SOMETHING AWESOME

SOMETHING AWESOME

A LIFE IN NEUROSURGERY

WILLIAM A. FRIEDMAN, MD

RADIUS BOOK GROUP
NEW YORK

Radius Book Group
A Division of Diversion Publishing Corp.
New York, NY
www.RadiusBookGroup.com

For more information, email info@radiusbookgroup.com.

First edition: February 2021
Trade Paperback ISBN: 978-1-63576-754-4
eBook ISBN: 978-1-63576-751-3

Library of Congress Control Number: 2020915557

Manufactured in the United States of America

10 9 8 7 6 5 4 3 2 1

Cover design by Charles Hames
Interior design by Neuwirth & Associates Inc.

CONTENTS

PREFACE

t's September 2020, and I'm going to tell you a story. It's a story about how highly trained, devoted individuals from disparate backgrounds can come together and, because of their devotion to their patients, strive to produce a good outcome. It doesn't always work (see chapter 10), but if the team is good, the outcome is usually good.

What's the most relaxing thing in your life? Although this will seem odd, for me it is doing complex neurosurgery. That's because I've been doing it for forty-five years, and I am blessed with incredible help, including my resident trainees, my partners, my staff, and everyone else (not least the folks who clean my operating rooms). And it's also because, unlike the unruly committee meetings I attended for years as chairman of the University of Florida (UF) Neurosurgery Department, in the operating room I am usually in charge. I tell my partners and residents frequently, "Thank God the brain surgery is so easy, because the rest of this will drive you crazy!"

The fact is, I am no longer chairman. On July 1, 2018,

after nearly twenty years as the second chairman of the UF Neurosurgery Department, I stepped down. My colleague and friend of many years, Brian Hoh, took over. He has done a *very* good job. Honestly, I like being ex-chairman. It has given me more time to do what I really like best, neurosurgery. And if I have a problem, I just complain to him!

September 2020 means that you, just like me, were trying to survive the worst pandemic since the 1918 flu that wiped out millions of people. Our country is reeling from over one hundred ninety thousand deaths (and this is almost certainly a gross underestimate), economic devastation, riots about police brutality toward blacks (the Civil War never ended for the white supremacists all around us), etc. The pandemic has exposed the gross weaknesses in our health-care system that have put minorities at a much higher risk of death from COVID (see chapter 19). But after a month of no elective surgery, we are back to full speed in the operating room. All patients are COVID tested. We, of course, wear masks. And we observe social distancing whenever possible.

Emergency/urgent neurosurgery never stopped. One night a patient presented to the emergency room. She had a one-week history of headaches. At home, she seemed to faint, but her family observed jerking movements in her right limbs. She was urgently transported to the UF/Shands emergency room. By the time she arrived, she was back to normal. A magnetic resonance imaging (MRI) scan showed a very large brain tumor, originating from the large vein that runs down the middle of the head (we call that the sagittal sinus). Portions of that very important vein were occluded by the tumor. Tumors that arise from this area are usually meningiomas. They are slow growing. That is why the patient was without symptoms until she had a seizure. A seizure is an electrical malfunction in the brain that frequently leads to jerking movements of the arms and legs, just as happened with this patient.

My partner, Dr. Greg Murad, was on call when this patient came in. Greg grew up in Vermont. His parents are both Spanish language professors at the University of Vermont. His brother is now chief of police in Burlington, Vermont. Greg attended med school at the University of Vermont. He came to us for neurosurgical training and was exceptional. During residency he met and eventually married Amy, who is the daughter of the most famous of all baseball umpires, Harry Wendelstedt. They have two wonderful daughters.

I offered Greg a faculty job and was thrilled when he accepted. Currently, he is our residency program director, a very challenging job. A superb neurosurgeon and a wonderful friend and colleague, Greg takes a lot of calls and was totally booked with cases, so he asked me to take this one. I was very happy to do so.

I don't usually worry much about neurosurgery, but this case concerned me. I could see that the tumor was very vascular (bloody) and that a lot of the blood supply was coming from vessels that normally supply the brain. I asked my partner, Adam Polifka, to do a blood vessel X-ray (called an angiogram) and to try to eliminate the vessels feeding the tumor by injecting material, called onyx, into them.

Adam is thirty-nine years old. Why would that matter? Well, my oldest child, Dan, is thirty-nine. So that must mean I am old, right? Well, I didn't feel old until I recently experienced a totally unexpected medical problem (see chapter 25). In any case, Adam trained in neurosurgery at the University of Maryland. He did an endovascular (treatment by injecting coils or other stuff into the arteries) surgery fellowship in Philadelphia. He is a great neurosurgeon and is also a great favorite amongst our trainees because of his teaching skills. Adam did the angiogram on this patient and injected onyx into some of the vessels supplying the tumor. It went well.

So, off we went to surgery. The neuro-anesthesiologist, a very valued partner, smoothly put the patient to sleep. I positioned the patient and applied a metal head-holder (called a Mayfield, named after a wonderful neurosurgeon from Cincinnati, my hometown). We then registered the patient's position to the surgical computer (called a stealth station). Using the computer, we outlined the anterior, posterior, medial, and lateral extent of the tumor. I then drew, with an ink marker, an incision that would encompass that tumor and a little more.

The patient was prepped (scrubbed with antimicrobials) and draped. Chief resident Will Carlton was my assistant that day. "Chief resident" here means that he was in his sixth year of neurosurgical training after medical school. Will is a graduate of the Virginia Military Institute and the Wake Forest University School of Medicine. He is from a military family. One of his distant ancestors knew Wilhelm Röntgen, the Nobel Prize–discoverer of X-rays, around 1900, and was one of the first to bring X-rays to the United States. Will is a major in the US Army and will be an army neurosurgeon after he completes his training with us. He is a superb doctor and surgeon. I love working with him.

Will and his assistant, junior resident (three years out of medical school) Kaitlyn Melnick, opened the skin. The scalp is very vascular, so we apply Raney clips to stop the bleeding. Then they used a drill to place several burr holes in the skull. Then, using a different power tool, Will and Kaitlyn sawed through the skull, starting at the burr holes, but continuing along the entire, predetermined line of incision. Once the skull was removed, the immediate problem was bleeding from the covering of the brain, called the dura. Although Adam Polifka had injected onyx into the vessels supplying the dura, and I could see it, the dura was still bleeding a lot. How to stop it? We simply incised the dura all the way around the tumor and coagulated the edges—bleeding stopped.

Here's the trick for removing this kind of tumor. It's usually benign. And it originates from the dural covering of the brain. So, once the skull is off, the job is to detach the tumor from its dural blood supply. We had already opened the dura over the top of the tumor and stopped the bleeding. Now we proceeded to rapidly detach the tumor from another dural source of blood, called the falx. The falx is a thick membrane that divides the two sides (hemispheres) of the brain. Once the tumor was detached from the falx, all that remained was to separate it, now with no blood supply, from its margin with the brain. That was the easiest part. Off the tumor went, in several large pieces, to the pathologist for microscopic examination.

One major thing was left. Remember that big vein down the middle of the head, the sagittal sinus? Well, it was full of tumor. So, we divided the vein in front of and behind the tumor and removed it. Then it was a simple matter of controlling bleeding and closing all of the layers that we had opened.

The patient awakened bright and alert, conversant, but with severe weakness on the right side. This was not surprising because of the brain manipulation required to remove the tumor. By the next morning, she was normal. However, the next day, she experienced repeated episodes of right-sided weakness and speech difficulty. So, what do we do when patients start to do poorly after brain surgery? First, we get an X-ray of the brain, called a CT (computed tomography) scan, to make sure there isn't postoperative bleeding. In this case, as is common, there was no bleeding.

The next thing we do is work with our neurology partners to make sure the patient isn't having more of those electrical brain malfunctions, called seizures. Our patient was hooked up to continuous brain wave monitoring and was, indeed, found to have seizures. This occurs in upwards of 25 percent of post-op cranial surgery patients who aren't doing well. With Neurology managing multiple seizure medications, the patient gradually recovered to normal. All was well. I have since seen her back in my office, and she's in very good condition.

What's this all about? Well, I hope this case illustrates

the intricate interplay of multiple caregivers, complex equipment, and true expertise in producing the best outcomes that we can currently do in the field of neurosurgery. This book is really about my decades-long journey to get here. How did I learn, often the hard way, to make the right decisions (see chapter 25)? How did I learn that every member of my team was so important (see chapter 24)? How did I learn about the pluses and minuses of health care in the United States (see chapter 19)? How did my patients and my own failings teach me humility over and over again (see chapter 16)?

Friends, please join me as I recount my journey in the following pages. A major reason for the success of this journey was the devotion of teachers, family, friends, and colleagues, but most importantly, it was because of my patients and their families. It has certainly been "Something Awesome."

WAF

EARLY DAYS | 1

My father, Jerry Marion Friedman, was a World War II veteran, having fought for six months in the Philippines prior to VJ day. He was then chosen, based on his height (6'2") and his army entry exam scores, to serve in General Douglas MacArthur's honor guard in Tokyo for a year. Upon returning home, he briefly attended Ohio State University on the GI bill, then enrolled in the University of Cincinnati law school. Upon graduating, Jerry returned to Dayton, Ohio, where most of his extended family had lived for decades. His mother, Jean, was the American-born daughter of a Lithuanian rabbi. His father, William Chaim Friedman, was the son of Lithuanian immigrants, who were in the "junk" business in and around Dayton.

One of the most notable events in my father's life was the sudden death of his own father, William Chaim, to a heart attack, when Dad was only twelve years old. Dad's mother had a total breakdown, and he was substantially cared for by his grandparents and other extended family.

Another notable event was his enlistment in the army at age seventeen, determined to fight for his country.

My mother, Phyllis Adele Kottler, was born in Nashville, Tennessee, to two more Lithuanian Jewish immigrants, Isaac and Belle Kottler. Grandpa Ike was initially an itinerant peddler but later opened a general store in Nashville. Grandma Belle, before marriage, worked in sweatshops to put her brothers through school. During the depression, Grandpa lost the store and required prolonged psychiatric hospitalization. They later moved to Dayton. Mom had two much older brothers, so she was the baby of the family. She went to school with my dad's younger brother, Bob, but then met my dad when she was only sixteen and fell in love. She graduated later from Miami University of Ohio. They married in 1952. I knew my Kottler grandparents as deeply kind and loving and simply adored them.

My dad eventually settled on working for the Prudential Life Insurance Company. In the fifties, he became the manager of the Queen City Agency in Cincinnati, Ohio. There, after skipping the sixth grade, I attended Deer Park High School, graduating in 1970. I then attended Oberlin College for three years before enrolling in The Ohio State University College of Medicine (then a three-year school). So, somehow, I wound up three years younger than my contemporaries. This was to have consequences.

One of the most notable events in my early life was my father's first heart attack when he was thirty-three years old. He had almost all of the risk factors we know about now: a bad family history, super-high cholesterol levels, a two-to-three pack a day smoking habit, and a sedentary lifestyle. I had just turned six and really just knew that Dad was going to be spending the summer at home with me, my mom, and my two sisters. I remember being sent away to live with my aunt Gertrude and uncle Julius, in Dayton. I loved staying in their big house and learning how to swim at their club. I also remember spending a lot of time with Dad learning my letters and sounds. By the time I started the first grade, I was reading well, which was relatively uncommon at that time.

Ten years later, when I was in high school, Dad had a series of further cardiac events, culminating in a visit to the Cleveland Clinic, where doctors were doing some of the nation's first cardiac catheterizations and coronary artery bypasses. I still remember him returning from that trip. I opened the door, and he just stood there and asked for Mom. He later told me that the fellow performing the catheterization kept repeating "impossible." After much time, a more senior cardiologist took over and completed the study. The result: inoperable multivessel coronary artery disease, left ventricular dysfunction, a left bundle branch block. In other words, get your affairs in order.

I quite vividly remember awakening from sleep in our small house to the sounds of my dad, moaning in the living room with crescendo angina. My mother tried to help him by rubbing his chest. Sometimes the doctor would stop over in the evening to give him a shot of morphine. I remember several hospitalizations and not knowing if Dad would survive. I remember my uncle Bob driving down at least once a week to take us out to dinner and try to help us. Somehow, Dad survived all of this. Although he remained on digoxin, long- and short-acting nitrates, and Coumadin for the rest of his life, he lived well into his eighties. But he was unable to return to work. My mom went back to school to get her teaching certificate. I remember her substitute-teaching my senior Latin class! The next year she went to work as a senior year English teacher at Sycamore High School. Of course, she still did all of the cleaning, cooking, and generally keeping the household functioning, as was the custom in those days. She loved being a teacher, and she loved being our mother. She loved Dad very much until her untimely death many years later.

In early 1973, I found myself interviewing for medical school. Almost always, the interviewers would ask, "Why do you want to be a doctor?" Strangely enough, I always struggled with the question. I talked about being inspired by my pediatrician or one of my parents' doctor friends. I don't actually remember talking about my family's deadly struggles with heart disease. Guess I just didn't want to think about it.

EDUCATION | 2

Early in my third year of college, I solidified my decision to become a doctor. I was aware that some medical schools were accepting "qualified" students after only three years of college. I asked my faculty advisor, Norman Craig, professor of physical chemistry, whether that was a reasonable plan. He had two physician brothers-in-law and wrote to both of them. One wrote back that medical school and residency took a very long time, and I might as well get on with it. The other wrote that leaving college was a mistake—I needed to learn more about life and become more mature if I wanted to be the best possible doctor. I remember he specifically said it was very important that I read and understand Alexander Solzhenitsyn's *Cancer Ward* if I wanted to take care of cancer patients (Solzhenitsyn, 1968). I decided to "get on with it."

Once at Ohio State, I immersed myself in the usual first-year courses—gross anatomy, biochemistry, and physiology. I really disliked dissecting the cold, stiff, formaldehyde-infused corpses. We moved on to microbiology, pharmacology, and, very importantly, for me, neuroscience. I absolutely loved neuroscience. Neuroscience includes aspects of anatomy, physiology, and pharmacology. But anatomy is what makes it so much different, clinically, from most other specialties. A good neuromedicine (neurology or neurosurgery) clinician can tell from a detailed neurological exam almost exactly where a lesion is located within the nervous system. Once the lesion is localized, careful perusal of the patient's history usually yields a list of likely diagnoses, the differential diagnosis. Then, appropriate imaging studies and other tests are ordered to confirm the diagnosis and suggest a course of treatment. The cold logic of neurological diagnosis remains, even in this day of modern diagnostic imaging, an irreplaceable and ever-stimulating part of neurosurgery. We will get back to this point in the coming chapters focused on clinical neurosurgical diseases.

At the beginning of my second year, we were afforded the chance to spend a day following a resident working with real patients. I was assigned to the gastroenterology service. I don't remember much about that day except the liver biopsy. We entered the patient's hospital room. As I watched, the resident prepped the patient's abdomen, injected a small Novocain weal in the skin, and then jabbed an impossibly long needle through the skin and into the patient's liver. The biopsy specimen was withdrawn, followed by an impressive amount of blood. I still remember my vision starting to gray out and constrict. I came very close to fainting and falling on my face during my first day on the wards!

Finally, our classroom studies were over, and we began the month-long clinical rotations that would occupy the rest of our medical school time. My first month was surgical subspecialties, and I was assigned to spend the first two weeks on neurosurgery. So, what did I know about patient care on my first day? Basically, nothing. I had done a few histories and physicals in my physical diagnosis course. But I had never started an IV, drawn blood, read an X-ray, scrubbed or gowned in the operating room, etc. I would learn all of this and much more over the next months. But that inaugural day, first thing, I found myself on neurosurgery rounds, led by chief resident Richard Dewey.

Dr. Dewey immediately drew my attention to a myelogram (an X-ray of the lumbar spine after the injection of dye) and asked for my interpretation. Honestly, I had no idea as to whether the myelogram was upside down or not! I had never even seen a chest X-ray. I had no answer for Dr. Dewey, but he had one for me—he thought I was an idiot. He seemed to have a desire to reinforce that view many times as I worked near him over the subsequent weeks. I don't remember him actually taking the time to teach me anything. I do remember his impatience and cruelty. He was a true asshole, one of several I would encounter in my future surgical career. I kept close to the junior residents and interns as much as I could. They welcomed me as a fellow traveler and taught me a lot.

My last encounter with Dr. Dewey was toward the end of my two weeks. He had assisted Dr. Hunt, the chief of neurosurgery, on an operation to relieve a severe facial pain condition called trigeminal neuralgia. The operation they performed was a very old one, developed by the founder of neurosurgery, Harvey Cushing. They made a small hole in the right temple on the side of the pain. Without opening the dura, they elevated the temporal lobe until they could see the sensory ganglion, which controls facial sensation (the trigeminal or Gasserian ganglion). Then they removed part of that ganglion and closed.

I stood next to Dr. Dewey in the recovery room, in front of a completely comatose and immobile patient. I thought I saw the patient move, but Dewey snickered at me and told me it was just the breathing machine. He and Dr. Hunt took the patient back to surgery, where they found a large hematoma caused by their failure to adequately coagulate the middle meningeal artery (a well-known hazard of this particular surgery). The patient died. I swore I would never have anything more to do with neurosurgery.

In the summer of my third and last year of medical school, I had pretty much made up my mind to pursue a career in neurology. In July, I got a call from the new chief resident of neurosurgery, Eric Zimmerman. Eric said he knew I was headed for neurology, but told me that Neurosurgery had a great program they were offering only to a few top medical students. I could do a senior clerkship with them during which I would carry my own call beeper and take every other night in-house call, just like the residents. It was an opportunity I could not refuse. In fact, I wound up taking call with Eric himself every other night.

This time I was ready. I could do a good neurological exam. I could write orders, draw blood, start intravenous lines, scrub, sew, and tie in the operating room. I was basically Eric's assistant for the entire month, as we rounded on a service of seventy-some patients, operated daily, and saw many, many emergencies. This was before the advent of CT scanning, so head trauma patients were evaluated by sticking a needle into the carotid artery, injecting dye, and taking a few X-rays. By studying the shift of the normal brain vessels, one could identify or rule out hematomas.

One night, Eric put the needle in my hands. I remember that they were shaking. I coauthored a paper with Eric and another resident—my first paper. I gave a slide presentation to the division, including the faculty, on a type of spinal cord injury called central cord. By the end of this rotation, I was convinced I wanted to be a neurosurgeon. I think I really just wanted to be like Eric Zimmerman. The Dewey-Zimmerman contrast is a compelling example of the profound influence that bad and good teachers can have on our lives. Mine was never to be the same.

THE ELEVENTH NERVE | 3

When I was a freshman medical student, I developed two small lumps, just below the skin, in my left neck. My doctor was concerned that they were swollen lymph nodes and might be something serious. So, I was sent to an ENT physician, Dr. Sidney Peerless, for an excisional biopsy. He removed them under local anesthesia—I was fully awake. During removal, my left shoulder started to twitch involuntarily. I had no idea why. I remember Dr. Peerless asked me if I was intentionally moving, and I said no. Well, the lymph nodes turned out to be small fatty tumors, called lipomas, which are completely benign. But I had some weakness and pain in the left shoulder area that took quite a while to resolve.

There are twelve paired cranial nerves that supply various muscles and organs of the head and body. The eleventh nerve is called the spinal accessory nerve. Its major component, unlike the other nerves, arises in the upper cervical spinal cord. Small rootlets leave the side of the cord and coalesce to form a nerve that ascends through the hole at the base of the skull called the foramen magnum. It, along with cranial nerves nine and ten, leaves the skull through a hole called the jugular foramen. It then travels to innervate two muscles, the sternocleidomastoid and the trapezius. The sternocleidomastoid is the principle rotator of the head. The trapezius allows people to shrug their shoulders.

One curious thing about the eleventh nerve is that it travels immediately beneath the skin in the posterior neck. So, surgeons doing biopsies in that area, if they are not careful, can damage the nerve. Dr. Peerless was somehow stimulating that nerve during my biopsy, leading to involuntary movement of the trapezius. The injury was mild and eventually resolved. But it isn't always so.

Many years later, I received a call from Ted Copeland, chairman of the Department of Surgery at the University of Florida. He had biopsied a cervical lymph node in one of his chief residents, Scott Rotatori. Scott came back to him, complaining of shoulder and neck pain. Sure enough, on exam, he had weakness of the sternocleidomastoid and trapezius. An electrical test called an electromyogram (EMG) confirmed the presence of an eleventh-nerve injury.

I later took Scott to surgery. We identified the two ends of a severed eleventh nerve. Unfortunately, the ends were too far apart to sew back together without undue tension. So, I harvested a small sensory nerve, called the sural nerve, from the side of his right ankle. I used the sural nerve as a graft between the two ends of the eleventh nerve. Using the operating microscope and sutures about the size of a human hair, I reconnected the nerve.

Nerves tend to regrow at about one inch a month. Sure enough, three months later, Scott was back to normal. Surgery for accessory nerve injuries tends to be successful for several reasons: First, it's a pure motor nerve. There are no sensory fibers that might regrow into motor channels. Second, the distance between the nerve injury and the target muscles is short. So the muscle can be reinnervated before it suffers permanent degeneration.

Even more years later, I was called by a general surgeon from my hometown of Cincinnati, Ohio. Dr. Edward Saeks had been a special friend of my family for many years. In fact, he had been in my mother's K-12 classes back when they were kids. When he was in college, and my dad was in law school at the University of Cincinnati, they roomed together for several years. Dr. Saeks had injured an eleventh nerve during a posterior cervical node biopsy. He was being sued. Could I provide any help? Sure, I could. I could recommend someone who could repair the nerve in Cincinnati. And I could provide testimony that our own chair of surgery had made a similar mistake. All turned out well.

As mentioned in other chapters, most neurosurgeons get into the field because they are fascinated by the complex, yet orderly organization of the nervous system. Understanding the precise function of brain areas and nerves can allow us to localize the lesion and propose a diagnosis, perform appropriate tests, and, ultimately, provide treatment. Here are some cranial nerve pearls:

Cranial nerve I mediates the sense of smell. It is frequently injured in anterior skull trauma.

Cranial nerve II subserves vision. The pattern of visual loss on exam can very precisely locate the lesion all the way from the eyeball to the occipital lobes of the brain.

Cranial nerves III, IV, and VI innervate the muscles that move the eyes. Cranial nerve VI is affected by increased intracranial pressure, leading to a lack of ability to move that eye laterally.

Cranial nerve V supplies sensation to the face. When compressed by a small blood vessel, it can lead to trigeminal neuralgia, a very painful disorder that can be relieved by surgery (discussed in chapter 10).

Cranial nerve VII moves the face. It is frequently intimately attached to benign tumors in the back part of the brain and requires much skill to preserve while removing such tumors.

Cranial nerve VIII gives us hearing and balance.

Cranial nerve IX innervates one small muscle in the throat.

Cranial nerve X, the vagus nerve, innervates the heart, the GI tract, and other organs.

You now know what cranial nerve XI does.

Cranial nerve XII innervates the tongue. Injury leads to atrophy of one side of the tongue.

There are dozens of patient stories to go with each of the dozen cranial nerves.

LONESOME TOWN— LETTERS FROM THE PAST | 4

There's a place where lovers go
To cry their troubles away
And they call it Lonesome Town
Where the broken hearts stay.
—Ricky Nelson, "Lonesome Town"

Leaving the Nest for Oberlin College

September 11, 1970

Dear Mom and Dad,

Well, I finally recovered enough composure to sit down and write a letter. After I finished talking to you today, I went to the library and worked on chemistry till nine. Then Stu and I went over to the Wilder (the Student Union) to play ping-pong as we've done the last couple of nights. Tomorrow I plan to sleep late (I'm tired) and spend the afternoon reading history. If I'm lucky, maybe I'll be able to play some tennis. Also, the Mummer's Show is tomorrow night, and I'm going to see it.

As of today, I've been to all my classes. Latin, like I told you, has only four students (that's something else I have to do). Chemistry is a larger but also interesting class. Math looks fascinating (but hard). Today I programmed a project titled A12593AN, FRIEDMAN. The first time it didn't work because I forgot a space on one of the fifteen or so computer cards! Stuart found it, though, and it worked. Actually, all I did was instruct the computer to make a running total of the odd numbers between one and sixty-five. It's not as easy as it sounds, though.

History's going to take some getting used to, but so does just about everything here. We picked up fresh linens yesterday. It's really very neat. (I taught Stuart how to make a hospital corner!) I bought just about everything I need, but I may buy another T-shirt or a gym suit. Tennis starts Monday. It looks pretty good.

Things are starting to get better. The shock of coming here is pretty great. It's not that there's anything wrong; it's actually very nice. But just when I had really become comfortable and happy in a lifestyle, well, here I am in another, different one. It's not hard to exist here. It's probably easier to learn here. But to learn how to live here, to be really happy and to lead a full life, that's the hardest thing I face. So, at times, when I think about the security, the true, restful peace, which often seems so elusive here but that I could almost always find at home—well, that's the essence of a sad, lonely kind of feeling.

But, like I said, things are getting better. As each day goes by it gets a little easier. I'll be talking to you soon. Miss you all.

Love, Bill

Leaving Medical School for UF

June 24, 1976

Dear Mom and Dad,

It seems like I write you a series of letters about every three years. I think that's because that happens to be the interval at which my life turns somewhat upside down, albeit temporarily. Anyway, I suppose it's better than no letters at all!

As you know, Chuck flew back to Cincinnati this morning. I must admit I had hoped he would stay longer. The prospect of six days before work starts seems more than a bit lonely at this time. I'll just have to make the best of it. We had a great time on vacation. Disney World was even better than Disneyland—I'm sure you'd like it too. The Hilton Inn at Riviera Beach was delightful. Between the tennis courts, pool, great beach, and excellent seafood, we had a time to remember.

Dad, I must say that the apartment couldn't be better! Now that the furniture is in place and everything is packed away, the place looks great. It's spacious, warm, and comfortable. The pool and laundry room are just outside the door.

It seems somewhat silly that, after such a nice vacation, sitting in a beautiful apartment and in the city of my own choosing, I should have any complaints. Yet I'm afraid that, even as a doctor and twenty-three years old, I'm still the same person who couldn't bear to stay away at summer camp. Part of my nature refuses to say goodbye to the pleasant past without a tearful struggle. I know that Gainesville will fast become my new home. But right now, I can't help but remember the security, friendship, and sense of well-being I knew in Columbus. The last few years of medical school were fine years—much better than anything I had known since I left home for Oberlin. As somebody said, "Every time I learn the answers, they change all the questions!"

The damned thing is that even though I intellectually realize that, with my friends scattered to the winds, even Columbus wouldn't seem the same—at the moment my emotions have gotten the better of me. I miss having good friends and peers to talk with about life and the happenings of the day. I miss having my family within an easy two hours. The sense of proximity was always a tremendous comfort.

In any case, I think it's good that you aren't coming down just now. I've got a lot on my mind and a lot of adjusting to do. I think in a month or so I'll be a new person. Or rather, I'll be the same person, but my environment will have changed.

You know, if family or friends or life weren't worth anything, then I wouldn't feel any remorse or regret at this time. It's these life changes that always make me realize (emotionally, not just intellectually) just how sweet and good and worthwhile my life has been and how grateful I should be for what I have. That's the real reason I'm writing all of this to you—to share that thought with you.

Love, Bill

June 29, 1976

Dear Billy,

We have your letter of the 24th and Mom and I were very moved by your expressions. To say that we understand your emotions at a time like this is really not enough and not very comforting. However, we do understand and vicariously are experiencing this time of turmoil and stress with you.

Your final paragraph really said it all, Billy. The fact that what you have, family and friends, so valuable and close, makes change difficult. Unfortunately, that is the price or other side of the coin involved with love and friendship.

However, I do have two observations, Bill. First—your family and close friends are always yours. That has not changed even though your residence has. Second—this change will most likely be the easiest of your life, because you will be with peers in the true sense of the word and also because of the very busy work schedule that you probably will already be engaged in by the time you get this ...

Let us hear from you soon.

Love, Dad

CHOOSING A | 5
TRAINING PROGRAM

I n the late summer of my senior medical school year, I set about finding my home for the next six years, the spot where I would do my neurosurgical residency training. Eric Zimmerman, my mentor, advised me to do an externship month at the University of California, Los Angeles (UCLA), where he had done his internship. William Hunt, the chief of neurosurgery at Ohio State, told me I should take a look at "young Al Rhoton's program" at the University of Florida. Both young Al and Bill Hunt had trained at Washington University in St. Louis under Henry Schwartz. Wash U was then regarded as the "cradle of neurosurgical chairs" because so many trainees had become chairs.

First, I went to Yale, where I stayed with one of my friends from Oberlin College. I took a train from New Haven to Boston to interview at Tufts. Upon boarding the train, I ran into two of my friends from high school, Mike Blum and Bobby Lovett. I hadn't seen them for years! I wound up sleeping on the floor of their apartment that night. I interviewed at Tufts, where Ben Stein was chair (this was shortly before he moved to Columbia). I remember sitting in the cafeteria with him as he asked me to list the common tumors of the posterior fossa. I came up with glioma and meningioma but couldn't remember any others. He was clearly not impressed.

My next trip was to Gainesville, Florida. I flew into Gainesville on Eastern Airlines and collected my bag under an open-sided shed. As the taxi left the airport, we passed a billboard that said, "Welcome to Gainesville, the other Florida." I thought that this, indeed, was unlike the South Florida beach destinations where my family loved to vacation. The next day I met the faculty, all four of them: Al Rhoton, George Sypert, Frank Garcia, and John Vries. I spent a little time with John Grant, whom I knew from medical school at Ohio State. He was then an intern in neurosurgery at UF. He was very busy, but let me know he liked UF.

I remember meeting with then-chief resident Arthur Day in Dr. Rhoton's lab. Art held a skull and asked me to name various holes at the base. I think I missed them all! Oh well. I was the number one student in my medical school class and was confident I could make up any knowledge deficiencies. I was very, very impressed with Dr. Rhoton. He had a gentleness and kindness about him that I hadn't seen in many of the surgeons I had met so far (except Eric Zimmerman). I thought he would make a great mentor.

A week after my visit to Florida, I got a call from Dr. Rhoton. He offered me a job. That placed me in a difficult position. I still had several interviews and was scheduled to do an externship at UCLA in November. I told him that I very much liked UF but couldn't in good faith accept an offer until I had finished those visits. He hesitated but then offered to wait. These days, residency spots are distributed through a computerized match. After interview season, the students submit a rank list of their choices. The programs do the same. That way students are guaranteed of "matching" at the institution highest on the list that wants them. So much better than playing chicken with department chairs.

On to Minnesota. I arrived there on Halloween, and it snowed all day. I spent most of that day sitting in the hallway outside the neurosurgery office, where Shelley Chou was chair. Two or three people spent fifteen minutes apiece with me. There was no tour, and no real organized attempt at recruiting. I headed to the airport and took a late afternoon flight to Los Angeles, where I was to begin my externship the next day.

The arrangements for the externship were interesting. Remember, this was back in the pre-cell phone, pre-computer days. I had made multiple phone calls to the UCLA neurosurgery office, requesting help finding a place to stay for the month. No help was forthcoming. So, I did what I'm sure I could never do today: I took a cab from the airport to the hospital ER. There, with my suitcase in hand, I asked them to page the neurosurgery resident on call. I explained that I was his new extern and asked if there was any place I could sleep!

Luckily, neurosurgery had a two-bed call room. The two

interns took call every other night. So, one bed was vacant. I took the bed and unloaded my suitcase into the dresser. I spent the next three weeks there. At first the intern's beeper going off every fifteen minutes was an issue, but after a few nights I never heard it. The chief resident gave me meal tickets, so I basically ate and lived in the hospital. The residents were terrific teachers. The service was small, about twenty patients. The chair, Eugene Stern, clearly liked the neurological exam a lot (like me) but didn't seem to care much for actual surgery. I liked UCLA. But not as much as Florida.

Toward the end of my externship, I made arrangements to fly to San Francisco for an interview at the University of California, San Francisco (UCSF). The night before my trip, I was on call. I remember a deeply comatose patient in the emergency room. UCLA had just installed its first CT scanner. The images were very grainy, but it looked like the patient had suffered a hypertensive intracerebral hemorrhage. I was up most of the night trying to get his blood pressure down to normal.

Come morning, I left for the airport and flew to San Francisco. I took the bus from the airport to downtown San Francisco and then walked quite a way to the hotel the UCLA residents had recommended, the St. Francis. I had a list of things to see in San Francisco—my interview wasn't till the next morning. I checked in around noon and decided to rest my eyes for a few minutes. The next thing I knew, it was 8 p.m.! The day was shot, but I certainly felt more rested. I wandered along the street outside the hotel and came across an interesting-looking restaurant, called

George Mandikian's Omar Khayyam. Inside, I sat at a long table with strangers and had a superb Armenian meal.

The next morning, I interviewed at UCSF. I remember one interview in particular, with Phil Weinstein. He asked me what I liked most about neurosurgery, and I told him I was fascinated by the way a careful neurological history and exam could reveal the location of the lesion and the most likely diagnosis. He said I should probably go into neurology, not neurosurgery!

On that day, one of my classmates, Michael Bowman, an MD/PhD candidate, also interviewed at UCSF. They clearly preferred him. That night, Mike and I ate dinner at Alioto's on Fisherman's Wharf. We went to the airport. He flew to Columbus. I flew back to UCLA. UCSF went on to offer Mike the job. He lasted six months as an intern, then quit.

On the way back to Columbus, I stopped at Washington University. I still remember watching neurosurgical grand rounds. The neurosurgical chair, Sidney Goldring, joined by a few other faculty, absolutely destroyed the chief resident as he was describing how he would handle a case. The junior resident who gave me a tour assured me that he would never come to Wash U if he had it to do over again. So much for the cradle of neurosurgical chairs. I called Dr. Rhoton and sealed the deal.

Two days after graduation, my dad put four new tires and a set of brakes on my car. I set out with everything I owned in the trunk for Gainesville. My best friend, Chuck Davidow, who was then at Harvard Law School, accompanied me on the trip. My father had a business interest in Orlando, so he had been able to scout out apartments in

Gainesville and rent one for me. He had found a great place, just a mile from the hospital, on a lake. I now had a one-bedroom apartment of my own.

I spent a few days reviewing my surgical textbooks and getting a sunburn by the pool. I got a short haircut. On June 30, all of the new interns met at William Pfaff's house for a welcoming reception. Dr. Pfaff, who was to be my internship mentor, was a general surgeon who had great warmth and personality. I noticed that the vast majority of my fellow interns also had new haircuts and sunburns!

INTERNSHIP | 6

Don't bend; don't water it down; don't try to make it logical;
don't edit your own soul according to the fashion.
Rather, follow your most intense obsessions mercilessly.
—Franz Kafka

Neurosurgical residency training has changed quite a bit since I did mine from 1976–1982. I've tried very hard to be a constructive part of that change. For now, let's go back to 1976.

The internship year, the first year out of medical school, was then a rotating general surgery year. I spent five months on general surgery at three different hospitals, including Shands, the Gainesville Veterans Administration (VA) Hospital, and the Lake City VA. I did one-month rotations on cardiovascular surgery, urology, orthopedic surgery, ENT, neurosurgery, and the emergency room. Most of that time, I took in-house call every two to three nights. Effectively, that meant I was usually working over one hundred hours per week. But so what? Everyone did it, and we viewed it as a definite sign of weakness to complain about fatigue.

My first rotation was cardiovascular surgery (CV). My first night on call, there were two cardiac arrests on the service. I called the CV fellow, Herb Martin, for help, but he assured me I would do just fine on my own. Both patients survived the night, not due to my ability, but due to the abilities of the ICU nurses and the more experienced anesthesia residents. I don't think I ever saw an attending physician in the hospital at night during my internship. Any and all issues were handled by the residents. There was a junior resident on call for all surgical services in-house who could help you but, again, it was a sign of weakness to call. I saw a lot of patients die that month.

The chief of CV surgery was George Daicoff. To my inexperienced eyes, he appeared to be a skilled surgeon but also appeared to have no interest in post-op care, which is critical to good outcomes in that field. I met my future wife, Ransom, that month. She was a pediatric cardiovascular surgery nurse clinician. I also became good friends with Herb Martin and Dick Brunswick (a junior attending), as well as the other residents on service.

General surgery rotations are a blur to me now. I bonded with the junior and senior residents who ran the services. We rounded twice daily, stayed in-house every two to three nights, and saw our attending surgeons in the operating room (OR) and once a week for Saturday morning rounds. In those days, academic surgeons made very little money, did a limited amount of surgery, and spent a lot of time on laboratory or clinical research projects. Nationally, it was fully accepted that residents would do most of the patient care, including all emergency surgery at night. The attending physicians and the hospital were expected to bill for the services rendered by residents. There was virtually no malpractice concern, nor did most patients expect to see the attending very often. I remember doing very simple procedures like hemorrhoidectomies, sebaceous cyst resections, appendectomy assists, etc., that I doubt had any real usefulness for a future neurosurgeon. I sure did learn how to work up a post-op fever!

At the Lake City VA, I was left alone from Friday afternoon till Monday morning as the surgical house officer. Basically, I was the only doctor in-house for all of the post-op surgical patients. One night, I was summoned for a cardiac arrest. I quickly performed my first-ever intubation, then started a central line, while the nurses did CPR. We found ventricular tachycardia (VTach) on the EKG and did an electrical cardioversion. The patient slipped back into VTach, we cardioverted again and administered lidocaine. We resuscitated him, but I don't believe he ever regained consciousness.

Back at Shands, I started my emergency room rotation. At night, the ER was staffed by a surgical intern, a medicine resident, and … no other physicians. I saw every manner of surgical patient and did my best to make a correct diagnosis and to call other surgical residents as needed. I remember calling Art Day (doing a second chief resident year) one night to see a compound skull fracture patient. Art took a look at the patient and asked me what I thought about that white stuff coming out through the fracture. It was brain!

Art whisked the patient off to surgery, and I went back to my backlog of patients. Another time, Art was seeing a patient and walked by as I was inserting a chest tube in a patient with a pneumothorax. "Way to go, Willy," he said. Art was to become my very best friend in the neurosurgery department for many years to come, another Eric Zimmerman, a true older brother figure.

On urology, I enjoyed working with junior resident Jorge Leal. One patient sticks in my mind. She had bilateral staghorn-shaped kidney stones. That means that most of the center of her kidneys was occupied by a large, stony, mineral deposit. This was causing renal failure. I watched the residents (the attending, Birdwell Finlayson, was a solid scientist but didn't really like surgery) do a procedure where they split the kidney in half, removed the large stone, and then sewed it back together. I was on call that night.

I checked on the patient, who was in the ICU, in the late evening, and she appeared to be doing well. When I made my pre-rounds (rounds before the whole group rounded), I found the patient severely hypotensive, tachycardic, and lying in a large pool of fluids that had exited the kidney through a drain and soaked her bed. My response was to yell like a maniac at the nurses for not letting me know a thing about her deterioration. Of course, this did the patient no good and permanently pissed off the ICU nursing staff.

The chief of urology, David Drylie, called me to his office and castigated me for my behavior. I remember thinking at the time that he should have been mad at the nurses, like me. They, after all, had made the mistake, not me! I also had to meet with my mentor, Bill Pfaff. I remember him nodding and saying, "You really take these things to heart, don't you?"

Remember the consequences of being three years younger than my contemporaries, mentioned before? I clearly had a high IQ but a low EQ. It would take years, and a lot of counseling from a variety of mentors, before I understood that everyone I was working with was trying to do the very best job they could. They sincerely wanted to help the patient and to help me. It took years for me, and neurosurgery as a field, to fully embrace the team concept that was to be so successfully embraced by aviation and other industries. To achieve maximum success, the environment must be "flattened" so that everyone on the team feels secure enough to speak out if they see something wrong. The imperious pilot or surgeon simply squelches the other team members' efforts, leading to poorer outcomes and a lot of unhappiness on all sides.

Anyway, I, and all those around me, survived the internship year. I was married to Ransom in June and began true neurosurgical training on July 1, 1977.

NEUROSURGICAL RESIDENCY | 7

To seek, to strive, to find, and not to yield.
—Lord Tennyson

B ack in the day, five years of neurosurgical residency training followed the one-year rotating surgical internship, for a total of six years of postgraduate training after medical school. Today, the rotating internship has been absorbed into overall residency training, and the total duration of training has increased to seven years post-med school. Assuming that one graduates from college at age twenty-one, doing med school and a neurosurgical residency gets you to age thirty-three. Then you are typically deemed ready to either join an academic neurosurgical faculty at a medical school or can go into private practice in a community setting.

For reasons mentioned before, I found myself starting residency having just turned twenty-three. I was now effectively apprenticed to the five UF neurosurgical faculty: Albert Rhoton, Frank Garcia, George Sypert, John Vries, and Arthur Day. Jack Maniscalco was also there during my intern year but left to go into private practice in Tampa. This was a very interesting and, for me, very influential group of people.

I will say the most about Albert Rhoton because he was my teacher, colleague, and friend for almost forty years. No one, other than my parents, has had more influence on the course of my professional life. Albert was born November 18, 1932, in rural Parvin, Kentucky, in a log cabin without electricity or plumbing. The midwife who delivered him was paid with a bag of corn. His early schooling was in a small two-room school that housed all eight grades. His mother was a teacher, although she held no degree. Nonetheless, Albert made it to Ohio State University.

It was during part-time work with groups of disadvantaged children while a student there that Albert decided to pursue a degree in social work. He noted in a later interview that all of his social work courses were well attended by the football players! Due to the influence of a spectacular teacher in physiological psychology, he decided to become a neurosurgeon and switched his major to pre-med. He flunked all of his initial exams and realized that he needed to stop working so many hours and spend more time studying.

Albert wrote his father, who was a wonderful man whom many of us were privileged to later know well, and his dad responded, "It does a boy good to go hungry." Fortunately, a friend was able to loan Albert some money. He got the extra study time and wound up with A's in all the courses. He went on to graduate number one in his medical school class at Washington University. After a two-year stint at Columbia in New York, Albert returned to Wash U for neurosurgical training.

After residency, he joined the Mayo Clinic faculty and,

in 1972, was recruited by Ed Woodward (the UF Chair of Surgery) to become chief of neurosurgery at the University of Florida. When he became head of neurosurgery at the University of Florida, there were two faculty members. During his tenure as chairman, Albert landed the first million-dollar donation in the history of the University of Florida system. He subsequently obtained funding for ten endowed chairs for research and education in cerebrovascular, pediatric, spinal, computer-assisted and stereotactic surgery, and microsurgery and neural regeneration. At the time of Albert's transition out of the chairman's position, his former residents, donors, and friends contributed more than two million dollars to be matched by another two million dollars from the State of Florida to complete the Albert L. Rhoton Jr. Chairman's Professorship in the Department of Neurological Surgery. He played a key role in the development of the McKnight Brain Institute, a six-floor building devoted to neuromedicine, which opened in 1999.

Dr. Rhoton's accomplishments in the areas of surgery, research, and training are legendary and Herculean. But much more than those great things, we must admire the man. As Osler said, and Dr. Rhoton endlessly demonstrated, "Happiness lies in the absorption in some vocation which satisfies the soul; we are here to add what we can to, not to get what we can from, life."

Dr. Rhoton said in a presidential address,

Our lives have yielded an opportunity to help mankind in a unique and exciting way. Our work is done in response to the idea that human life is sacred, that the brain and nervous system are the crown jewels of creation and evolution, and that it makes good sense to spend years of our lives in study in order to be able to help others. The skills we use are among the most delicate, most fateful, and to the layman, the most awesome of any profession.

During an incredible interview in the University of Florida History of Medicine series, Dr. Rhoton was asked the following hypothetical: "If God came to you and said that if you worked as hard as you could through college, medical school, and neurosurgical training such that you could save one and only one life, would you do it?"

Dr. Rhoton responded, "Absolutely, yes."

In the brilliant movie *Schindler's List*, Steven Spielberg recounts the story of the Schindlerjuden, the hundreds of Jews saved by the actions of Oskar Schindler during World War II. In gratitude, one of them made, as a present for Schindler, a gold ring from extracted dental fillings. On it, he inscribed an ancient Talmudic saying, "He who saves one life saves the world entire."

Of course, Dr. Rhoton and his many students have saved not just one life, but thousands. Thousands have lived because Dr. Rhoton lived.

Richard Selzer, a Yale surgeon, wrote,

I do not know when it was that I understood that it is precisely this hell in which we wage our lives that offers us the energy, the possibility to care for each other. A surgeon does not slip from his mother's womb with compassion smeared upon him like the drippings of his birth. It is much later that it comes. No easy shaft of grace this, but the cumulative murmuring of the numberless wounds he has dressed, the incisions he has made, all the sores and ulcers and cavities he has touched in order to heal. In the beginning it is barely audible, a whisper, as from many mouths. Slowly it gathers, rises from the steaming flesh until, at last, it is a pure calling, an exclusive sound, like the cry of certain solitary birds, telling that out of the resonance between the sick man and the one who tends him there may spring that profound courtesy that the religious call Love (Selzer 1976).

Unfortunately, we lost Dr. Rhoton to cancer several years ago. But we who loved him, and the whole world of neurosurgery will never forget him.

Francisco Garcia-Bengochea was born in Cuba. He did his neurosurgical training at Columbia University and cared for Johnny Gunther Jr. (discussed in chapter 11, "Glioblastoma"). He returned to Havana and became the premier neurosurgeon, not only in Cuba but for referrals from Central and South America. His wife was an heir to the Bacardi fortune. Life was good until Castro came to power. The Garcia family left Cuba with nothing and settled in Kansas, where Garcia practiced neurosurgery at the university. His brother, an engineer, lived in Gainesville, so the family eventually moved.

Garcia became the go-to neurosurgeon for this new medical school in the era before Al Rhoton arrived. The division, at that time, was run by Lamar Roberts, a graduate of the Montreal Neurological Institute. Unfortunately, he was a hopeless alcoholic. Garcia rescued him and the division until Rhoton arrived.

Frank Garcia was the consummate gentlemen. I never once saw him raise his voice in anger. He was calm and cool during difficult surgeries. He was kind and gentlemanly. He retired after my chief resident year. His son, Javier, is a very successful private practice neurosurgeon in Jacksonville, FL.

George Sypert was one of Rhoton's first recruits. He had trained at the University of Washington in Seattle and had a superb background in both clinical neurosurgery and basic neurophysiology. George was a fearless, if somewhat erratic, neurosurgeon. He was probably the one faculty member most willing to let residents actually do surgery under his supervision. In this sense, he was a good teacher of neurosurgery. He also had an amazing partnership with a neurophysiologist named John Munson. George and John had a beautiful neurophysiology laboratory, continuously funded by the National Institutes of Health (NIH) and the VA, as a result of their steady scientific output.

After a year of residency, I knew I wanted to stay in academics. I asked Dr. Rhoton how best to prepare, and he referred me to George. Of course, George thought the best option was for me to spend a year in his lab! He was right. Sypert helped me prepare a predoctoral NIH fellowship application that was funded. I wound up spending fifteen wonderful months in the lab. Our research focused on basic spinal cord physiology, using a cat model. I learned animal surgery and anesthesia. I learned how to perform intracellular neuronal recordings and how to use spike-triggered averaging to detect and record electrical potentials from a single sensory axon going into a single neuronal body. By the end of the experience, I had learned a great deal about electrophysiology, which I was later able to translate to the operating room environment.

In the OR, George was nervous and, sometimes, manic. In the lab, he was totally relaxed and became a real friend. Using what I learned under his tutelage, I was able to write another grant to the NIH, which funded my research for my first five years on faculty.

George was also my mentor in terms of focusing me on clinical research areas, all of which became important in my later career. He became one of the early neurosurgical adopters of new spinal instrumentation techniques. He sent me to learn a brand-new lateral discectomy technique from a neurosurgeon in Miami. This led to several of my first publications. He also connected me with Peter Heilbrun at the University of Utah and got me going in the very early days of CT-guided stereotactic surgery. Finally, he recommended that I look into a new tumor treatment called radiosurgery. More about all of this later.

When I was a young faculty member at UF, George got divorced from his second wife, Nancy. He later met and married a pediatric neurosurgeon, Joy Arpin. Joy wanted to join us at UF. But we had significant concerns about her. George and Joy left for private practice in Ft. Myers, where they were very successful. George was angry, and rightly so. He had done very much for me, and I had not helped him.

John Vries had trained at the Medical College of Virginia under Don Becker. John was a pediatric neurosurgeon. He was a brilliant man but a mediocre surgeon. He taught me how to do a twelve-minute ventriculoperitoneal shunt, but not a lot more. He left to become chief of pediatric neurosurgery at the University of Pittsburgh. Later, he became one of their IT leaders. Computer science, I think, was his true love.

Art Day was the youngest of the faculty. As such, he naturally had the greatest affinity for the residents. Art was a great teacher. We all looked forward to his X-ray rounds on Wednesday at the VA, even though he was sometimes an hour late. He was extremely personable and charismatic. I greatly enjoyed working with him in surgery and in the clinic. At neurosurgical meetings, we shared a room several times. We played duplicate bridge every week when I was in the lab. We also played tennis and shared a love for Gator sports. I spent time in his office every day after I joined the faculty, talking about neurosurgery and life in general. Art was instrumental in getting me appointed to the Congress of Neurological Surgeons Executive Committee which, ten years later, led to me becoming president of that organization.

As long as I remained in the little brother role, Art was a terrific friend. When I started "growing up" and achieving clinical, academic, and leadership success, Art wasn't so happy. With the inevitability of a Greek tragedy, Art and I, in 1998, found ourselves competing for the job of department chairman. I got the job. Art never got over it. He eventually left UF to pursue his career goals elsewhere. I still miss Art.

Of all my teachers, Dr. Rhoton was the most demanding. During that time, we had about fifty patients in the hospital. The chief resident met with a senior resident, a junior resident, and an intern to make rounds around 5 a.m. We then had a one-hour conference, from seven to eight. At eight, we either went to the OR or started on patient care floor work. The entire team waited until the chief resident was out of surgery, then began rounds. This could be late evening, depending on how the day had gone. Then we began again at 5 a.m.

The chief resident, pretty much alone, communicated with the faculty on their patients. He was expected to know every detail. Of course, knowing every detail on fifty patients was impossible. And the fatigue was impressive. But that's the way it was.

As mentioned before, I was away from patient care for fifteen months in Sypert's lab before I returned to start my chief residency. I was rusty. One day in the OR, I found myself re-draping the microscope three times because I had forgotten the details of the setup. A week later, I got the dreaded voice page, "Call 2-2548." That was Dr. Rhoton's private office number. He wanted to see me.

Behind closed doors, Dr. Rhoton was very angry because I had not discharged a VIP carpal tunnel patient on rounds instead of after rounds. I apologized and told him I was still learning the ropes after my research rotation. He explained that the ropes, from now on, would involve me calling him every morning before going to surgery and every evening after completing rounds, without exception. So, for the next three months, I found myself calling the chairman, frequently in the late evening, awakening him to discuss his patients. He was always pleasant, and we never really had a problem again. Eventually, he told me I could stop calling.

JOBYNA WHITING'S TALE | 8

Joby Whiting wrote this essay while chief resident at UF.
She is now in practice in Miami, FL. I include this with permission.

Mrs. X arrived dead. It was the middle of a Saturday night call, and I was on with my chairman, Dr. Friedman, which always adds a certain amount of tension to an already fraught ordeal. I don't remember exactly what I was doing when the phone rang. The junior resident in-house with me was on the other end. "I've got two new ones to tell you about," he started, in an apologetic tone.

I immediately tried to focus on his monologue, searching for the inevitable buzzwords of significance that would be embedded somewhere in a seemingly useless amount of minutiae. With increasing seniority, I have become one of the people who doesn't always evaluate a patient primarily. Indeed, I often find myself being "presented" with a more junior resident's synopsis of a patient's story and neurological examination. I have been somewhat surprised by how difficult it can be to follow and make sense of these presentations, which often seem to emphasize everything except the pertinent details. On multiple occasions, I have realized that I can hear the resident's voice, but that I have stopped listening and cannot remember the last several things spoken, in much the same way that I can get to the end of a paragraph of text and realize I have no idea of what I have just read. In those instances, I can't help wondering if my attendings feel the same way when I present patients to them, or do they, with time, learn to recognize patterns of information regardless of the context in which it is displayed.

On this particular night, the junior resident started with Mrs. X: "I've got a 53 year-old woman who was the driver in a motor vehicle accident. She was stationary at a red light when she was struck by a pickup truck. Interestingly, the drunk driver of the pickup is my second consult, but I'll get to that later."

I shrugged away my irritation at this breach in presentation protocol and focused in on his continuation of Mrs. X's tale: "EMS reports that she was unresponsive at the scene with a GCS (Glasgow Coma Scale) of 3, whatever that means. She was intubated in the field and required prolonged resuscitation prior to arrival at our ER. They started to code her again, right after I got to her. The quick exam I got showed bilateral blown pupils, no corneals, no gag, no movement to pain. I think she's brain dead. I guess they'll scan her when she's stable, if she survives that long."

"Where is she now?" I asked.

"In the unit," he replied. "They'll call me when she's stable."

"OK. What's the next one?" I started to move toward the

ICU. Perhaps trauma surgery and Critical Care Medicine could stabilize Mrs. X in the time it took me to hear about the second consult. At any rate, a patient like this needs to be seen right away. My junior resident was very capable, but the responsibility is mine to ensure that we aren't missing something in a critically ill patient. Every move I make at the hospital occurs in the context of a continuous background of slight anxiety that I might be making a decision based on an erroneous assumption. I imagine it to be similar in a way to how a hockey goaltender lives, with the constant possibility of something dangerous and unseen suddenly getting by from the periphery.

"You're gonna love this," he replied. "Mr. Y is a twenty-eight year old male who was apparently sitting at home drinking all night. He got hungry and decided to go get something to eat in his pickup truck. He then proceeded to smash into Mrs. X's car as she was sitting at a red light. We got called because radiology saw a left C6 superior facet fracture. Head CT is negative. On exam, he's amnestic to the event. His GCS would be 15, except he's totally drunk, and his motor and sensory exam appear to be intact. We've got him in a collar, and I think we just need to let him sober up to get a real strength exam. He's up on 10-trauma."

"Okay. I'll look at him after I see Mrs. X. I'm just getting to the unit now—why don't you meet me down here?"

Mrs. X was pretty clearly dead. She had no brainstem reflexes on exam, and her head CT showed diffuse subarachnoid hemorrhage, particularly concentrated at the cervicomedullary junction. Reconstructions of her C-Spine CT confirmed my suspicion of atlantooccipital dislocation (AOD), and complete lack of intracranial blood flow on CT angiogram reinforced the overwhelmingly convincing clinical picture of brain death.

My junior resident showed up and I launched into a mini-lecture about AOD, and the clinical and radiographic findings associated with the disease process. I'm not always clear how welcome this sort of didactic is, given the typically late hour of occurrence and the crippling workload shouldered by junior neurosurgery residents on call, but I do it anyway. I really can't help it. In this case, I love the disease, and am always excited to see an example, although this is somewhat troubling considering the enormously high associated mortality.

Later in the morning, I spoke with Mrs. X's family. It's always a weird experience to tell someone that their loved one is dead; combining that information with an attempt to explain the logistics of brain death, and to convince desperate people that their loved one is truly gone in spite of a beating heart. So many people want to believe in the possibility of a miracle.

In this instance, I found myself in a small, awkward conference room with Mrs. X's husband and young adult daughter and son. Her husband took the news with unusual peace and composure. I was surprised, and slightly relieved. I asked if they would like the company of a chaplain or the like.

Mr. X smiled and replied, "I am a minister. There are four more in the waiting room. Thank you anyway." He then asked that I come out to the waiting room and explain things to the rest of the family.

I agreed easily and found myself in a room of about 10 concerned looking people. I was shocked to hear an unreserved wail erupt from an elderly gentleman whom I believed was Mrs. X's brother upon hearing my news. I had been lulled into a false sense of security by Mr. X's calm demeanor. I watched her brother rock back and forth, crying and angrily asking, "Why, God, why?" over and over, and was reminded of stories of sackcloth and ashes from the Old Testament.

Two women ran to the man and hugged and comforted him—he remained outwardly oblivious to their ministrations, and seemed almost to reject them. I watched their concerned faces and wondered slightly at their ability to become lost in this man's distress in the face of the personal grief I assumed they must certainly feel at the loss of Mrs. X. It quickly became clear that my presence was superfluous, and I excused myself to move on to the next consult.

Entering Mr. Y's room was a curious experience simply because I knew he killed Mrs. X. I didn't know what to expect, really. Nothing in my life prior to residency prepared me for what to think about interacting with people in the middle of these types of horribly life-altering tragedies. Mr. Y was indeed neurologically intact. He avoided eye contact and stared at the wall. He was guarded closely by a small young woman who sat by his bedside with a large wedding set prominently displayed on her hand. She was aggressive and far more interactive than Mr. Y. She answered questions directed toward him in a manner that had hints of both defiance and desperation. There were no police in the room.

I had only told Mrs. X's family of her death a few minutes previously, and it occurred to me that this tenacious little woman (Mrs. Y?) couldn't know the details of how bad the situation was, but she was certainly sharp enough to know that this man of hers was in serious trouble.

Later in the day, I returned to discuss final treatment recommendations with Mr. Y. Again, he was minimally involved in the interaction. This time, a woman several decades older than the previous one was hovering over his bed. She was his mother, and she looked anxious and distraught. The room was oppressively quiet. I glanced from Mr. Y's expressionless face and dead eyes to the pinched, apprehensive face of his mother. I thought of the angrily frightened look on his tiny wife's visage. The whole scene was reminiscent of a DH Lawrence short story I read in college called "The Odor of Chrysanthemums." In it, a woman and her mother-in-law explore feelings of anger, grief, and guilt in the context of the death of the woman's husband, killed in a mining accident. Although the details did not fit exactly, I was struck by the enormous and conflicted influence Mr. Y's actions were having on the lives of these two women.

For days, I found myself wondering at the night's surreal contrasts. A single event can elicit the troubling excitement of learning first-hand about a rare but well-described neurosurgical injury at the cost of a woman's life and her family's happiness; that same event renders a young, healthy man's life effectively over for the foreseeable future, if not permanently. His actions leading to said event reverberate in a devastating manner in the lives of two women to whom he is intimately linked. No wonder I have a glass of wine when I get home from work.

BAND OF BROTHERS | 9

We few, we happy few, we band of brothers. For he today
that sheds his blood with me shall be my brother; be never
so vile. This day shall gentle his condition. And gentlemen in
England now abed shall think themselves accursed they
were not here, and hold their manhoods cheap whiles any
speaks that fought with us upon Saint Crispin's day.
—Henry V, Shakespeare

Neurosurgical residency is an intense, anxious time. Our residents are frequently the brightest of the bright. But nothing in medical school can really prepare them for the high-stakes, high-pressure world of neurosurgery. First, they have to acclimate to the sheer number of hours of work. In the old days, one-hundred-hour workweeks were common. In 2006, the Accreditation Council for Graduate Medical Education (ACGME), the governing body of all US residency programs, limited the number of work hours to eighty hours per week, with at least one full day a week off.

As the UF Health Neurosurgery program director, I embraced these reforms because I had found the unlimited hours to be very fatiguing. Doctors don't do their best work when they are tired, and I was usually very tired, especially as chief resident. My schedule that year was as follows: Meet the other residents at 5 a.m. and make group rounds on the entire service, finishing in time for our daily 7 a.m. educational conference. Once a week, I was directly responsible for running the conference. Then off to the operating room until all of the cases were finished. Then meet the group again for rounds. If the OR ran late, these rounds could be midevening. Then work up the pre-op patients for the next day's surgery. Then home for a few hours of sleep. Unless I was on call, which I was every other night. Then I would inevitably be called by the in-house resident to come see floor or ER consults, usually multiple, frequently leading to very little or no sleep.

This routine makes even the most even-tempered (and that wasn't me) residents cranky. At its worst, it totally distorts our relationship with our patients. We all went to med school to help people, right? But if every beeper page or phone call about a patient makes you even more desperately tired, you begin to merge into the "patient as enemy syndrome." The work-hour reforms were intended to produce improved patient outcomes. That hasn't really happened (another story). But the reforms have tremendously improved the quality of residents' lives. I think they have also led to many more women entering the field, which is very good for neurosurgery.

Another inevitable aspect of neurosurgical training is that young doctors are constantly finding themselves in clinical situations where they are not quite sure what to do. This produces much anxiety. There is just so much to learn. Yes, they can always rely on their senior resident colleagues and their attending physicians to check them and guide them. But eventually they have to start making more and more decisions on their own. This is part of the graduated responsibility apprenticeship aspect of medical education. This anxiety is at its worst when actually learning how to do surgery. I found this part of neurosurgery the most draining during my early years after finishing residency, when I no longer had that supervisory safety net.

The combination of fatigue and stress generally leads to very close friendships between fellow residents. It's a bit like joining a fraternity or, perhaps, a military unit. I made lifelong friendships with five residents. I will say a few words about each of them.

I was extremely fortunate that UF Neurosurgery recruited Richard Jackson the same year they recruited me. Richard was a tall, athletic graduate of the University of Oklahoma. He was bright, capable, friendly, married, and mature. Over the years, he and his wife, Christie, became very close to me and my wife, Ransom. Richard and I were never competitors or rivals. We were friends who tried to help each other out whenever we could. His calm approach to problems and his superb interpersonal skills were a constant, helpful reminder to me that I needed to get much better in both areas.

One night when Richard and I were chief residents, I was so sick that every time I tried to get out of bed, I nearly fainted. Of course, I was on call, and, of course, the junior resident, Jim Menges, called me to see an emergency consult. I just couldn't do it, and I called Richard. I called him very reluctantly because he was just as tired as I was. He graciously told me not to worry and took care of everything for the remainder of that night.

Richard had a Prindle catamaran, which he liked to sail on nearby Lake Santa Fe. On several occasions he invited me to help him race the boat. We both donned wet suits. He was the captain, and I was the crew. My job was to hang over one of the hulls in a trapeze attached to the mast so that he could get one hull out of the water. My weight would counterbalance and prevent the boat from turning over. On at least one occasion, we turned the boat over multiple times. I finally got so tired from righting the boat and getting back on board that I couldn't do anything but hang onto the hull. Richard simply reached down, grabbed me by the neck of the wet suit, and lifted me with one hand back on board. Like I said, he was strong.

Richard went on to have a very successful career in private practice neurosurgery in Dallas. We enjoyed meeting at many subsequent national neurosurgery meetings. When he was president of the Texas Neurosurgical Society, he invited me to be honored guest. I last saw Richard at a dinner celebrating my stepping down after twenty years as chairman of UF Neurosurgery. He's still the same great guy I met in 1976.

As mentioned in a previous chapter, one of the residents a year ahead of me was John Grant, a fellow Ohio State University medical student. I didn't spend a lot of time professionally with John—since he was only one year ahead of me, we were rarely together on the neurosurgical service. But he and his wife, Jeannette, became very close friends of ours. My wife and I took many vacations with them, both during and after residency. We spent many holidays together at their house or ours in Gainesville.

When John finished, he went into private practice in Cocoa Beach, Florida. Later, he moved to Norfolk, Virginia. Every summer, for many years, John, Jeannette, and their three boys would spend one to two weeks with Ransom, me, and our three kids at St. Augustine Beach, Florida.

Unfortunately, John crashed and burned. He became enamored of another woman. Believe it not, she talked him into writing fake narcotic prescriptions that she would fill and sell on the street. Eventually, he was caught and had to plead guilty to a third-degree felony to avoid going to jail. I don't think John realized that this would automatically place him on the Medicare/Medicaid do-not-pay list, which in turn led to loss of hospital privileges. Despite many efforts, he was never able to practice neurosurgery again. The last time I saw him, he was still trying to get a presidential pardon.

The other resident one year ahead of me was Dick Lister. Dick came to UF from the University of Illinois College of Medicine in Peoria, IL. He was married with one child. Dick managed to do a great job of balancing his neurosurgical residency duties with his family responsibilities. That meant that he didn't have a lot of time to socialize with the residents, like me, who didn't have kids. We enjoyed a very cordial relationship, nonetheless. When he finished, he went back to Peoria, where he pursued a very successful career at his med school alma mater.

About ten years into my chairmanship, Dick called me

and said that he was looking to leave Peoria and wondered if I knew of any opportunities around the country. I thought for a minute and said, "Why don't you come back to UF?"

Shortly before moving to Gainesville, Dick told me that he had just been diagnosed with early Parkinson's disease. I told him that was absolutely not a problem. Dick came as chief of our VA Service, our residency program director, and associate chair. He was a godsend to me at a time in my career where I really needed a capable senior leader to help me run and grow the department. Dick was a fount of great ideas to whom I will always be grateful. After eight years, Dick retired and still lives in Gainesville. As he says, we are "brothers from different mothers, and our father was Al Rhoton."

Two years ahead of me were two remarkable people, each of whom became like an older brother as well as a great friend:

Tom Lansen was a University of Wisconsin med graduate. He initially became a psychiatry resident but quickly decided to switch to neurosurgery. So, Tom, his wife, and young daughter, Nora, moved to Gainesville. Tom was an Eric Zimmerman sort of senior and chief resident. He made the hard work of our daily lives fun. We spent a lot of time together taking care of neurosurgical patients, and our families spent a lot of time together socializing in our limited off time. We also enjoyed traveling together to neurosurgical meetings.

During my third year of residency, we found ourselves at the Congress of Neurological Surgeons meeting in Washington, DC. That year our boss, Al Rhoton, was president (as I was to be many, many years later). The president hosts a number of social events, including the Honored Guest Dinner, and the president's reception. Unfortunately, after one day at the meeting, I found myself not feeling so good. I started having shaking rigors and chills, followed by high fever. Then I would feel fine for about four hours, and it would start again. I asked Ransom to buy a thermometer. When I took my temperature, it was 105 degrees!

Let me assure you, it doesn't feel good to have a fever that high. Bottom line, although I tried to attend as many of the scientific sessions as I could, I didn't make it to the social events. Ransom went and told me later that Dr. Rhoton was quite unhappy that I wasn't there. She thought he believed that I was hungover! Anyway, Tom was there, and though he and all my other doctor friends (and I) failed to make the diagnosis, he was very solicitous of my health. They managed to get me on the plane home. Ransom drove me directly from the airport to the emergency room. A chest X-ray revealed the culprit, pneumonia. I started antibiotics and felt tremendously better by the next day. I took one day off work. While at home, I received a call from Dr. Rhoton, who had heard I had pneumonia. He told me, "I'm sorry I thought what I thought."

After graduation, Tom pursued a very successful practice in New York City and Westchester County. Tom remains one of the most charismatic people I've ever met. I love being around him.

Bruce Woodham was born in Chipley, Florida, and grew up in a family where no one had ever been to college. He came to the University of Florida as an undergrad. For some reason, he only applied to one medical school, UF, and was shocked when he didn't get in. He scrambled to find an alternative and wound up attending medical school in Belgium. He and his new wife, Mary Jo, found themselves in a country where neither one spoke the language (the school was in the French-speaking part of the country). Bruce later told me that, at the beginning, it would take him an hour to translate one page of his textbooks. However, he rapidly mastered basic French. He told me that it took about a month for him to start dreaming in French, and then he knew he had made it! He excelled in school and came back as a surgical intern at the University of Iowa. Then he came to the UF neurosurgical residency at the same time as Tom Lansen.

Like Tom, Bruce became a close friend and mentor. Off duty, we shared a love of scotch, steak, and rock and roll music. Bruce went into private practice in Dothan, Alabama, after finishing the residency program. I can easily remember my sadness when Bruce and Tom left. They were my best friends at the time. Ransom and I threw a huge party for them at my house that went on until the wee hours. Honestly, I got so drunk my hand would no longer hold my scotch glass, which dropped to the floor several times. The next day, I told Mary Jo Woodham that my hair hurt.

The next year was the time I spent in George Sypert's and John Munson's lab. One Saturday (yes, I worked every day even though it was a lab year), George came in and told me he had some very bad news. Bruce had been involved in an automobile accident and wasn't expected to live. I went home, packed a small bag, and immediately drove to the hospital in Dothan, about four hours away. Bruce was not doing well. He had substantial pelvic fractures and was short of breath, on oxygen. I drew the first blood gas he'd had since entering this so-called trauma center. It confirmed poor oxygenation. His vital signs were marginal, with a high pulse and borderline blood pressure.

I reviewed all of the X-rays and spoke several times to the general surgeon in charge. My conclusion was that they were not capable of successfully managing this kind of trauma. I called my old advisor, Dr. Pfaff, and asked him whether we should transfer Bruce to the University of Florida. He told me that since I was the physician on the scene, I would have to make the decision. So, I asked Bruce's partner, Bill Silvernail, who was a retired army reserve colonel, to see if he could get us helicopter transport. Helicopter transport was very unusual in those days. Sure enough, an army chopper landed on the roof of the Dothan hospital. I stuffed a paper bag with drugs and supplies for the journey, and off we went. I had never been on a helicopter before and didn't know how loud it would be. I could not take a blood pressure or even communicate by voice with Bruce.

As we approached Gainesville, they handed me a headset. The pilot said that the navigational beacon at UF was off, and he was lost. I looked down and could see I-75. I told him to follow the highway south. I then recognized the turnoff for the hospital. We turned right, and the helipad was in sight. Bruce went immediately to the ICU, where he remained for the next month.

Mary Jo stayed with Ransom and me for the next month. She was a wreck. So was I. I couldn't concentrate on anything except Bruce. I spent a lot of time in the unit with him. And the nurses called me day and night for any concerns that Bruce had about his care. He not only survived, but he went back to Dothan and continues to prosper as the go-to neurosurgeon in that area. This whole, somewhat surreal experience was a bit life-changing for me. I remembered that Talmudic saying, "He who saves one life saves the world entire." Well, I saved Bruce's life, and he went on to save hundreds more in his own practice. I felt that if I never accomplished anything else, I had received a great gift, the opportunity to save a best friend, and to feel that my life had a definite purpose.

TRIGEMINAL NEURALGIA | 10

t's called the suicide disease. Trigeminal neuralgia is a severe facial pain disorder. It is characterized by episodic, lightning-like stabs of pain on one side of the face. The pain is frequently brought on by touching the face, chewing, or brushing the teeth. It is frequently mistaken for some kind of dental disease, so many patients have had teeth extractions or root canals before they make it to a neurologist or neurosurgeon. It is usually relieved by a drug called carbamazepine. But, in many cases, drug therapy becomes ineffective over time or leads to intolerable effects like drowsiness or unsteady gait.

Early pioneers of American neurosurgery like Harvey Cushing and Charles Frazier successfully controlled patients with refractory trigeminal neuralgia by removing part of the trigeminal sensory ganglion, under the temporal lobe. It's basically the same procedure I saw William Hunt and Dick Dewey perform when I was a medical student. This procedure usually produced excellent long-term pain relief but at the price of permanent facial numbness. This led, in some cases, to ulceration of the numb cornea (an outer lining of the eye). Some patients, unpredictably, find the numbness very unpleasant. That's called anesthesia dolorosa.

About the time I was starting my residency, a neurosurgeon called Peter Janetta, building on observations of other neurosurgeons, came up with a theory to explain trigeminal neuralgia. Dr. Janetta observed that such patients usually had a small artery, typically the superior cerebellar artery, in direct contact with the trigeminal nerve as it exited the part of the brainstem called the pons. He found that he could relieve the pain, without permanent numbness, by dissecting the artery away from the nerve and placing a small sponge in between the nerve and the artery. This procedure is called microvascular decompression (MVD) or the Janetta procedure.

Later, Janetta observed that the same type of microvascular compression of the facial nerve could produce an intractable twitching disorder of the face, called hemifacial spasm. He revolutionized the treatment of these diseases (trigeminal neuralgia and hemifacial spasm) by making a simple observation. Initially, he endured much skepticism and criticism. But gradually his view became the new normal in neurosurgery.

My boss, Al Rhoton, had been trained to do another type of procedure for trigeminal neuralgia. In this procedure, the patient is briefly anesthetized. Then, using X-ray guidance, a small needle is inserted through the face into the trigeminal sensory ganglion. Using radiofrequency current (hence the procedure name, radiofrequency lesion or RFL), the tip of the needle is heated to about eighty degrees centigrade for about a minute. This procedure, popularized by a Harvard neurosurgeon named William Sweet, basically does, in fifteen minutes, what Cushing and others did in a much longer, riskier, open operation. The patient is left with facial numbness, but the pain is gone. About 50 percent of the time, the nerve will eventually regrow, and sensation returns, as does the pain. One simply repeats the fifteen-minute procedure if that happens.

Dr. Rhoton was initially skeptical of the Janetta procedure. But he rapidly became convinced and starting doing both RFLs and MVDs while I was in training. When I joined the faculty, I started doing them as well. When Dr. Rhoton wound down his clinical practice, I began doing all of the trigeminal neuralgia surgeries, now numbering about one hundred and fifty cases per year. We generally do the MVD on younger patients in good health and reserve RFL for older patients who might not tolerate a longer procedure under general anesthesia. We use RFL exclusively for another type of trigeminal neuralgia that occurs in patients with multiple sclerosis (MS). In this group, the pain is not related to microvascular compression but rather to an MS lesion in the brainstem.

A surprisingly small number of neurosurgeons treat trigeminal neuralgia. Given the fact that most patients are thrilled to be free of this horrible pain, that may seem surprising. But there are several confounders to overall patient satisfaction:

First, remember that this is a diagnosis made solely from taking the patient's history. There is usually no neurological abnormality on exam. An MRI may or may not show the offending artery or vein. So correct diagnosis is dependent on getting an accurate history from the patient, who is often in great pain and/or on drugs that cloud a person's thinking. In recent years, patients have already been on the internet, and they know exactly what questions are likely to be asked. All patients with facial pain who come to see me are absolutely convinced that they have trigeminal neuralgia. In fact, a lot of them don't.

There is a group of patients, typically younger women, who have a constant aching, burning pain in the face that is not responsive to carbamazepine. They have had a lot of dental and medical treatments. They are desperate for relief and view the neurosurgeon as their last, best hope. But we know from experience that this type of pain, called atypical facial pain, is not responsive to surgery. The most unhappy patients in my practice are the ones who I tell I cannot help with surgery because they don't have trigeminal neuralgia. Very frequently, despite my best efforts to explain, they believe I am wrong. They simply will not hear that they are not candidates for surgery. They hear, instead, that I won't help them. I would say that, as a general rule, that applies to patients with other potential neurosurgical problems, like back pain. They don't like hearing that they won't get the magical surgical cure.

Second, as with any kind of surgery, "stuff happens." Despite performing thousands of these procedures, I still have an occasional horrible result. Mrs. M was a healthy middle-aged woman with classic trigeminal neuralgia. I met her and her husband in my Thursday outpatient clinic. She was no longer responding to carbamazepine and was losing weight because eating brought on her pain. I reviewed the surgical options and explained the risks and benefits in detail (a legally and ethically required process called informed consent). Like many patients, she wanted to go ahead with surgery the next day.

We took Mrs. M to the operating room the next morning. After she was anesthetized, my resident and I placed her in the lateral position (on her side) so we could easily access the area behind her left ear. I shaved a small amount of hair and prepped her skin. The resident placed the surgical drapes and made a two-inch incision behind Mrs. M's ear. We used a drill to place a nickel-sized bone opening at the junction of two large venous drainage sinuses. We then opened the dura. The operating microscope was draped and moved in.

Using the microscope's superb lighting and magnification, I gently retracted the upper edge of the cerebellum and drained spinal fluid until the brain was relaxed. I then followed a pathway, outside the cerebellum, down to the petrosal vein. I coagulated and divided the petrosal vein, allowing the trigeminal nerve's point of exit from the brainstem to be clearly visualized. Sure enough, the main trunk of the superior cerebellar artery was compressing the nerve. I mobilized it and placed a sponge between it and the nerve. The resident closed, the patient awakened normally and was returned to the postoperative recovery room.

That evening, Mrs. M started complaining of a worsening headache. Her blood pressure rose to dangerously high levels. Because these patients often have headaches after surgery, the resident on call treated her with pain meds. He did not effectively control Mrs. M's blood pressure or move her to a higher level of nursing care. The family became frantic, and eventually, the resident ordered a CT scan. At this time, Mrs. M was drowsy, and the scan showed a hematoma, not in the surgical site but within the cerebellum near it. The resident didn't call me but instead called my partner, who was on call. They took Mrs. M back to surgery and did a decompressive operation without removing the hematoma. I found out about this the next morning.

I took Mrs. M back to surgery and, going through the original incision, removed the hematoma. But it was too late. She never regained consciousness and died a week later. A woman with everything to live for had come to me for help and, instead, had died. The family, with whom I spent a great deal of time, was, by turns, angry, then grieving. And thus began the process that occurs every time I have a bad result: relentless self-doubt and self-loathing. You veer into imposter syndrome where, for a time, you believe that you're not really a good neurosurgeon, that you are entirely unworthy. Bad results are especially hard on young neurosurgeons because they haven't had time yet to develop skills that they truly trust. As we care for the unfortunate patient and family, we must remember to also care for the distraught doctors, nurses, and staff who have failed.

Most catastrophes in medicine, like most aviation accidents, are not due to one event. They are, rather, due to a series of events, each one providing a missed opportunity. We call this "lining up the holes in the slices of Swiss cheese." In this case, a well-intended resident got caught in a cognitive trap—because all of the post-op MVDs he had thus far seen had done well, he was slow to believe that this patient wouldn't. Then he called a partner who was unfamiliar with the surgery instead of calling me. Why? Maybe he didn't want to disturb me. Or worse, maybe he was afraid that I would be mad—remember that flattening of the environment thing? We reviewed all of this at our departmental complications conference and changed a number of things for the better. Until the next time.

GLIOBLASTOMA | 11

I believe that man will not merely endure: he will prevail.
He is immortal, not because he alone among creatures has an
inexhaustible voice, but because he has a soul, a spirit capable
of compassion and sacrifice and endurance.
—William Faulkner

As my career progressed, I became more and more interested in treating brain tumors. Benign brain tumors, like meningiomas and schwannomas, can require a great deal of skill to safely remove, but can frequently be cured with surgery alone. Malignant brain tumors are, unfortunately, another story. The most common tumor that begins in the brain is called a glioma. These tumors are called primary brain tumors because they start in the brain. Other malignant tumors, which spread through the bloodstream from cancers elsewhere in the body, like lung or breast cancer, are called metastatic brain tumors.

Gliomas are traditionally divided into four grades. Grade I tumors, called pilocytic astrocytomas, occur in children and are often curable. Grade II tumors, called low-grade astrocytomas, occur in young to middle-aged adults. They have a five- to ten-year overall survival rate from the time of diagnosis. Grade III tumors, occurring in older adults, are associated with shorter survival, eighteen to twenty-four months on average. Grade IV tumors, called glioblastomas, are the most common gliomas and are the worst. Average survival is twelve to fifteen months.

So, what's the problem? Why can't we cure these tumors? Why have the results of treatment remained so stagnant for so long? There are many reasons, but the primary problem is that these tumors grow microscopically, a long way into normal brain. Now, elsewhere in the body, one can sometimes take a large margin of normal tissue around a tumor in order to attempt a cure. Not so in the brain. Taking normal tissue will frequently lead to disabling loss of neurological function, like paralysis, visual loss, speech difficulty. So, surgery is used for two purposes. The first is to establish the tissue diagnosis by harvesting tumor tissue for the pathologist to review. The second is to remove as much tumor as can safely be taken. The gold standard is called gross total resection. But even gross total resection inevitably leaves a large amount of microscopic infiltrative tumor that will rapidly grow.

After surgical resection, patients with glioblastoma are usually treated with radiation therapy. Radiation therapy focuses high-energy X-rays on the tumor bed plus a margin of about one inch. The treatments are usually given once a day, Monday through Friday, for six weeks (thirty treatments). Radiation's primary effect is to damage the DNA of dividing cells, leading to cell death. Since tumor cells divide rapidly and normal brain cells don't, the tumor is selectively killed, to a degree. For many reasons, some cells are able to escape the effects of radiation and lead to a tumor recurrence.

Also included in routine post-op treatment of glioblastoma is a once-daily, oral chemotherapeutic called temozolomide. Many years ago, a medical oncologist named Roger Stupp proved that the combination of radiation and this drug consistently produced about three more months of survival than radiation alone. So now the combination of maximum safe surgery, followed by six weeks of radiation with concomitant temozolomide, is called the Stupp protocol.

John Gunther, a distinguished writer, chronicled his son's struggle with a glioblastoma in a book first published in the 1940s. The book, *Death Be Not Proud*, should be read by every neurosurgeon. Listen to Gunther's words as he tries to find meaning in Johnny Jr.'s tragedy:

All that goes into a brain—the goodness, the wit, the sum total of enchantment in a personality, the very will, indeed the ego itself—being killed inexorably, remorselessly, by an evil growth! Everything that makes a human being what he is, the inordinately subtle and exquisite combination of memory, desire, impulse, reflective capacity, power of association, even consciousness—to say nothing of sight and hearing, muscular movement, and voice and something so taken for granted as the ability to chew—is encased delicately in the skull, working there within the membranes by processes so marvelously interlocked as to be beyond belief. All this—volition, imagination, the

ability to have even the simplest emotion, anticipa-
tion, understanding—is held poised and balanced in
the normal brain, with silent, exquisite efficiency.
And all this was what was being destroyed. It was, we
felt, as if reason itself were being ravaged away by
unreason, as if the pattern of Johnny's illness were
symbolic of so much of the conflict and torture of the
external world. A primitive to-the-death struggle of
reason against violence, reason against disruption,
reason against brute unthinking force—this was what
went on in Johnny's head. For others, I would say that
it was his spirit, and only his spirit, that kept him
invincibly alive against such dreadful obstacles for so
long; this is the central pith and substance of what I
am trying to write, as a mournful tribute not only to
Johnny but to the power, the wealth, the unconquer-
able beauty of the human spirit, will, and soul (Gunther, 1953).

Neurosurgeons are afforded a great gift, the opportunity to help patients who are desperately in need of help.
They and their families often welcome us with open arms
into their lives. They trust us with their lives. They will give
us their friendship and their love if we are open to them.
Caring for patients with incurable diseases is a profound
privilege. It is a privilege, however, that is tainted with
equally profound sadness.

Ms. W was a thirty-two-year-old emergency room nurse
when she presented with a seizure and was found to have
a posteromedial right frontal mass. I performed a

craniotomy and gross total resection of a low-grade mixed glioma. She underwent postoperative radiotherapy. Shortly thereafter, Mrs. W returned to work full time. Subsequently, she quit her emergency room job, formed a brain tumor support group, and devoted most of her time to writing patient support literature and helping other patients with brain tumors. Three years later, she was found to have a recurrence. On repeat craniotomy, she had a frank glioblastoma. She began chemotherapy and later died.

This patient was a physically beautiful woman. She was also vivacious, intelligent, and caring. She was unfailingly positive and optimistic, regardless of what her MRI scans seemed to show. She never lost hope.

When I last saw her, Mrs. W's external beauty was marred by hair loss and Cushingoid symptoms from steroid therapy. She and I both knew that time was short, and there was little more that medicine could offer. Nonetheless, we talked at length about her plans for the future. She thanked me for all my efforts. I thanked her for allowing me to be her physician. When we hugged each other at the end of her visit, we knew we would not meet again in this world.

EVOKED POTENTIALS | 12

During my residency, I was fortunate to be able to spend a year learning basic neurophysiology techniques from George Sypert and John Munson. As I finished that year, with their guidance, I worked on a new NIH grant proposal to use those techniques to look at spinal cord injury in a cat model over a five-year period. Initially, I heard back that my grant was scored too low to get funding. One day later, my father called. "Congratulations, Bill. You got your grant!"

I was happy, but also puzzled, and maybe a little irritated that my father, who was a retired insurance executive, knew about my grant before I did. "Dad, how do you know?"

Well, it turned out that his friend, a Cincinnati ENT physician named Sid Peerless (the doc who operated on my neck), was on the NIH Council. The council passed final judgment on funding grants in the marginal score range. So, Sid called my father with the good news, and my father called me!

On July 1, 1982, at age twenty-nine, I became an

assistant professor of neurosurgery at the University of Florida. I became occupied with the triple mission of academic neurosurgeons: operating, teaching, and doing research. The research part initially followed the script of my grant. We created spinal cord injuries in cats, watched over them for several weeks, then did experiments looking at excitatory and inhibitory connections (called synapses) in single spinal cord motor neurons. I'm sure this might have led to some valuable basic information about changes in basic neurophysiology after spinal cord injury. But I rapidly found out that I didn't like making cats paraplegic (paralyzed in the legs), even for a short period of time.

I had done some reading about a neurology testing technique called evoked potentials. This test involves a stimulus, such as a small electric shock over a peripheral nerve, a click in the ear, or a flash in the eye, and the recorded response over the scalp. The test involved many of the same neurophysiological techniques I had learned in the lab. The very small evoked response on one stimulus was swamped by the background electrical activity of the brain (the EEG). If you repeated the stimulus hundreds of times, the background noise averaged out to zero, but the evoked response added up in one direction. This test had been used for some years in neurology circles, mainly as a test for multiple sclerosis.

One or two centers (mainly the University of Pittsburgh) had begun publishing reports about using this technology in the operating room. This was long before the day when this equipment was commercially available. So, I took my neurophysiology equipment from the lab, mounted it on a rolling cart, and went off to the operating room. I hired a technician, Didi Gravenstein, who was fresh out of college. We discovered that we were indeed able to reliably monitor two pathways on patients undergoing neurosurgery under general anesthesia. First, we could stimulate a nerve in the leg or arm and record the brain somatosensory evoked potential from the scalp. Second, we could stimulate the ear with clicks, and record the brainstem auditory evoked potential. Why was this important? Well, if you can monitor a pathway during surgery, you can tell the surgeon whether anything he is doing is harming the pathway, sometimes enabling him to take corrective action.

My partners provided me with enthusiastic support. Drs. Sypert and Day both did aneurysm surgery. Aneurysms are small blisters that arise on brain blood vessels. If they rupture and bleed, they can be deadly. Back in the day, the only treatment was open surgery to place a small metal clip across the neck of the aneurysm. If the clip is slightly misplaced, it can occlude a normal blood vessel, leading to a stroke. We found the somatosensory evoked potentials could reliably predict whether many of these brain vessels were compromised, giving the surgeon an opportunity to reposition the clip.

My boss and, now, partner, Al Rhoton, did a lot of surgery for trigeminal neuralgia. As discussed in a previous chapter, the microvascular decompression operation involved moving a compressive blood vessel off the trigeminal nerve. The eighth nerve (the nerve of hearing) is very close. Too much retraction on the brain or too low a position of the retractor can damage the eighth nerve, leading to unilateral deafness. We found that we were able to monitor the eighth nerve with brainstem auditory evoked potentials. Again, the surgeon had ample opportunity to reduce or readjust retraction and avoid nerve injury.

Over time we found many more applications for evoked potentials, including scoliosis surgery, aortic surgery, and peripheral nerve surgery. I began to collate our results and write papers on our experience, which were published in neurosurgical journals. This led to many invitations to speak on the topic at national meetings. We also began teaching three-day courses in Gainesville, so that other neurosurgeons could come and learn how to do this. Then we began hosting annual meetings. Soon I was known as an expert on intraoperative evoked potential monitoring. Over the course of ten years, I supervised the monitoring of four thousand five hundred patients. So began the academic research side of my career. Evoked potential monitoring is now routine in all neurosurgical operating rooms around the world.

We also found that evoked potentials could be used as a diagnostic adjunct in the diagnosis of brain death in intensive care patients. One day my tech and I rolled our neurophysiology equipment up to the pediatric intensive care unit. There we stood before a beautiful, blond four-year-old. He had been totally well until the previous week when he had contracted the flu. His mother treated him with baby aspirin as was routine at the time. But instead of getting better, the boy became rapidly worse. When his mother brought him to the emergency room, he was barely responsive. This little boy had contracted a disease that we don't see anymore because we now know that the interaction of the flu virus with aspirin can sometimes produce something called hepato-cerebral or Reye's syndrome that is characterized by fulminant liver failure and severe swelling of the brain. Didi and I did somatosensory and brainstem evoked potential testing. Neither were present. I looked at the poor, distraught, weeping mother, and I thought of my own young son, Daniel.

When I was a resident, I thought for a long time that I wanted to be a pediatric neurosurgeon. I am so glad I am not.

IS THERE A DOCTOR IN THE HOUSE? | 13

I suspect that all physicians, at some point during their career, will be called upon to deliver emergency medical care away from their usual places of practice—their offices or their hospitals. I can recall five times when I have been involved in such incidents.

In 1976, when I was a surgical intern, I was driving home. About a block ahead of me, I saw a car plow into a motorcycle rider and speed off. I pulled up to the curb beside the comatose rider. A pediatrician I knew also pulled over. I made sure the victim was breathing and that his spine was protected. Soon an ambulance pulled up. I started a large-bore intravenous line. I rode the ambulance back to the UF emergency room with the man and turned him over to my friends on neurosurgical call. I regret that I do not remember how he did.

In 1986, my friend and colleague, Frank Bova, and I were looking to implement a radiosurgical system at the University of Florida (see chapter 15). One summer afternoon, we were waiting in line to board a plane at the

Gainesville airport, bound for Boston, to visit two radiosurgical pioneers, Ken Winston and Wendell Lutz. I happened to be looking out the window just as a flash of lightning came down, striking the Eastern Airlines jet and then the baggage handler who was next to it. He immediately collapsed to the ground, and it started to rain heavily.

I ran out to the tarmac. The man was pulseless and not breathing. An ICU nurse I knew also came to the rescue. I started mouth-to-mouth respiration while she did chest compressions. Mouth to mouth, which I had never done before and haven't since, is remarkably personal. The man had a mustache. And he tasted heavily of tobacco. But, so what? We did cardiopulmonary resuscitation (CPR) for what seemed like a very long time before the emergency team arrived. They whisked him off.

I went ahead and boarded the plane, soaking wet, and Frank and I went off on what would prove to be a very eventful visit, leading ultimately to the establishment of the University of Florida radiosurgery system. The patient did not make it.

Florida is the state with the highest level of lightning-related injuries, due to the frequency of thunderstorms and the density of the population. In any given year, some two million lightning strikes occur, or twenty per square mile. This leads to about ten deaths per year. Lightning hits cause cardiac and respiratory arrest, burns, concussive trauma, and paralysis. The treatment is attempted CPR.

Years later, I was on a flight with my family, going from Denver to Atlanta, after a week of skiing. About ten rows up, prior to takeoff, a man started complaining of severe chest pain. The call went out, "Is there a doctor in the house?" It seemed to me that about a third of the passengers stood up! Well, it was the end of a ski week. Several of the docs were intensive care experts, so I wasn't needed. The patient was taken off to a local hospital, and our trip went on.

In 2014, my Acura Legend of twenty-plus years finally died. I bought the car I had wanted since I was sixteen years old, a Chevrolet Corvette Stingray. Part of the purchase included a three-day driving course at a short track about fifty miles west of Las Vegas. So off I went. When the course ended, I joined my youngest son, David, for a couple of days of fun in Vegas. Then I boarded a flight for home. Two hours into the flight, the call went out. This time, I was the only physician to respond. I was called back to see a man who had passed out in his window seat. He was morbidly obese and was clearly wedged into that seat and buckled in with a seat-belt extender.

I examined the man. He was comatose, with pinpoint-small pupils, poor eye movement, and minimal response to pain. I thought he probably had a brain bleed. His wife was an anesthesiologist. They lived in Tampa, Florida. They had just spent five days in Vegas with their family celebrating the man's seventy-fifth birthday. The wife said he had a great time and seemed fine when they boarded the plane. She assumed he was sleeping but eventually realized she could not wake him.

I soon recognized the limits of medical care on an aircraft. There was no way I could get the man out of his seat to a supine position. Listening to his heart and even getting vital signs was difficult due to the noise. Eventually, I was able to determine that his vital signs were stable. I advised the captain to divert as soon as possible. I probably spent more time trying to comfort the wife than doing anything useful for the patient.

We landed in Birmingham, Alabama, instead of Atlanta. It took a very big, strong fireman to lift the man out of his seat to a stretcher in the aisle and off to an ambulance. I don't know how he did, but probably not well. But he had just had a great five days with his family, and he basically died in his sleep. Is that all bad?

Fast-forward to 2016. My wife and I have two children and two grandchildren in London, England. We were traveling back from London to Atlanta, after a great visit. About four hours out of London, the call went out again. This time it was an elderly English gentleman who was coming to visit his dying brother in the States. He had chronic pulmonary disease and used oxygen at home. He had no oxygen on the plane, and because the plane is pressurized only to eight thousand feet, was feeling very short of breath.

The airline attendants were great. They provided me with excellent equipment to take the man's vital signs and measure his oxygen levels. The oxygen levels were low. We started oxygen, and he immediately improved. I told him that there would be an ambulance waiting for him when we landed. This provoked an unexpected response: "Please, doctor, I have no insurance and will be bankrupted by your system. Just let me go to my brother."

Well, we had no choice. Off he went in the ambulance. I hope he had a good reunion with his brother and got away from our rapacious billers.

STEREOTAXIS | 14

Stereotaxis means to touch in three dimensions. The concept has been revolutionary when applied to brain surgery. In the early part of the twentieth century, many neurological diseases had no effective medical treatment. Parkinson's disease, for example, with its progressively disabling tremors, rigidity, and slowness of movement, would have no effective drug therapy until the 1960s when L-dopa was discovered. Many severe psychiatric illnesses awaited the development of psychoactive medications. And some severe pain problems could not be controlled well with existing narcotics. What if a lesion could be made in the appropriate brain pathway, bringing some control to movement disorders, pain disorders, and psychiatric disease? It turned out that such lesions were usually in deep brain areas. The trick, then, was to be able to accurately target that area. Hence, stereotaxis.

So how does stereotaxis work? One needs to convert the brain's anatomy into a set of x, y, z coordinates. First, you attach a frame, usually a metal ring, rigidly to the patient's skull. In practice this can be done by inserting four small pins, under local anesthesia, to anchor the ring. Then you perform a radiographic procedure to identify internal brain coordinates. Then, using basic trigonometry, you calculate how to introduce a small probe through the skull and brain, to the target point.

In the early days of stereotaxis, before CT and MRI scanning, "indirect" targeting was used to identify targets. Air was injected through a small skull hole and via a catheter into the fluid-containing cavities of the brain, called ventricles. The anterior commissure (AC) and the posterior commissure (PC), which form the anterior and posterior border of the third ventricle (a small fluid cavity in the middle of the brain), were identified. The location of the target was indirectly determined based on a brain atlas that showed the location of the target in relationship to the AC-PC line.

Irving Cooper, a neurosurgeon, made an interesting discovery, accidentally, which revolutionized the treatment of Parkinson's disease. He was performing a procedure called a pedunculotomy, where part of the motor pathway to one side of the body is cut. This produces tremor relief at the price of significant weakness. During this procedure, Cooper inadvertently damaged the anterior choroidal artery. The pedunculotomy was aborted. To his surprise, the patient awakened with relief of many of his Parkinson's symptoms.

Now, purposefully sacrificing the anterior choroidal artery can, in some cases, cause paralysis, so that in and of itself is not a practical treatment. But the anterior choroidal supplies blood to the part of the brain called the globus pallidus. It turned out that lesioning the globus pallidus could relieve Parkinson's without causing paralysis! The era of stereotactic surgery for Parkinson's disease took off. Cooper later switched to a different target, the ventral lateral thalamus, which seemed to do more for tremors. Soon, hundreds, then thousands of patients were getting surgery for Parkinson's disease.

The history of stereotactic treatment for psychiatric disease is a lot cloudier. Egaz Moniz, a Portuguese neurosurgeon, found that lesioning the frontal lobes could calm patients with severe psychiatric illness. In 1949, he won the Nobel Prize in medicine for the invention of cerebral angiography, a method for visualizing the blood vessels of the brain. A neurosurgeon, James Watts, and a neurologist, Walter Freeman (a student of Moniz), performed the first frontal leukotomy (cutting white matter fibers) in 1936. They worked together for a decade and performed over two hundred procedures. Freeman, without Watts' knowledge, started doing a transorbital lobotomy by inserting an ice-pick-like instrument, under local anesthesia, through the roof of the orbit and into the frontal lobe. With a sweeping motion, the white matter pathways were cut. Watts objected that only a neurosurgeon should do brain surgery, but Freeman went his own way.

Freeman traveled the country and performed some four thousand lobotomies. He never wore a mask or gloves during these procedures. Many of these patients were severely disabled for the remainder of their lives. The case of Rosemary Kennedy (sister of JFK), amongst others, led to widespread criticism of this procedure. In the 1950s, Thorazine, a new drug, was developed, and this led to much more effective medical treatments.

Clearly, the Moniz-Freeman procedure did not use stereotactic guidance, but other psychosurgical procedures did. Lars Leksell, the Swedish neurosurgical giant, and Jean Talairach, a French neurosurgical pioneer, used their own stereotactic devices to target the anterior part of the internal capsule (another deep part of the brain) for patients with intractable obsessive-compulsive disease (OCD). Bilateral cingulotomies were proposed as an alternative to lobotomy in the 1940s and were first performed by British neurosurgeon Hugh Cairns for OCD and intractable depression. These procedures are still used today in a small number of centers around the world.

OCD is a relatively uncommon, but severely debilitating psychiatric disorder. Patients with OCD become entrapped by ritualistic behaviors that they cannot control. For example, a patient might feel compelled to wash his or her hands fifty times a day, even to the point of self-mutilation. A patient may not be able to go through a doorway without repeating a phrase dozens of times. Tragically, OCD patients are aware of their problem, but cannot control it. Today, stereotactic treatment for OCD involves two newer methods. The first is radiosurgery, which, as detailed in another chapter, involves focusing hundreds of radiation beams on a brain target. The most common target remains the anterior internal capsule, but the radiosurgical lesions are made noninvasively on an outpatient basis. Another approach, which has proven quite successful, involves deep brain stimulation (DBS). More about DBS below.

The entire field of stereotaxy underwent a revolution in the 1980s when computed tomography (CT) imaging became available. CT allows the brain to be directly imaged. At the University of Utah, a medical student (Brown), a neurosurgeon (Roberts), and an engineer (Wells) developed a CT-compatible stereotactic frame. Now one could directly image the AC and the PC, eliminating the need for ventriculography and complex calculations. But, more importantly, using CT, brain tumors could be imaged. Now stereotaxis could be used to treat anatomical lesions, as well as functional targets.

In 1983, I traveled to Utah to meet Roberts and Wells and watch another of their colleagues, Peter Heilbrun, perform a stereotactic biopsy of a deep-seated brain tumor. Soon, we had Brown-Roberts-Wells (BRW) frame number 33 at the University of Florida. Over the next ten years, I performed a number of stereotactic firsts in Florida— biopsies, DBS for intractable pain, brachytherapy (the insertion of radioactive pellets into brain tumors), as well as others. This became a new focus of my academic career. I wrote multiple papers, gave a number of talks at national and international meetings, and ultimately worked with my colleague, Frank Bova, to refine the computer technology needed to guide these procedures.

When MRI became available, the details of normal and abnormal brain anatomy became very much better than provided by CT. CT and MRI stereotactic guidance became the basis of two new neurosurgical revolutions.

The first, radiosurgery, involves stereotactically focusing hundreds of radiation beams on a brain target and is the subject of the next chapter. The second, DBS, has largely become the mainstay of modern treatment for Parkinson's disease, tremors, and OCD if they become refractory to medication.

DBS involves the stereotactic insertion of wires (electrodes) into deep brain targets like the thalamus and the subthalamic nucleus. These wires are usually placed bilaterally and are connected to pacemaker-like batteries under the skin. DBS is remarkably effective in the treatment of many movement disorders. It is also applied to smaller numbers of patients with intractable depression, OCD, Alzheimer's disease, and other brain diseases.

One of my students, Kelly Foote, who is now a professor in the UF Health Neurosurgery Department, and his colleague, Michael Okun, now chair of UF Health Neurology, run one of the largest DBS programs in the world. It is one of the greatest achievements of UF Health overall.

RADIOSURGERY | 15

A fool with a tool is still a fool.
—Grady Booch

n 1985, my mentor, George Sypert, came back from a meeting and told me about a new neurosurgical treatment, called radiosurgery, that had been developed in Sweden. He thought I should look into it. Radiosurgery is a technique where hundreds of small beams of radiation are all focused on one spot, say a tumor, in the brain. It is an outpatient treatment because the beams actually go through the skull to the target. The type of radiosurgery most commonly used today was originally conceived by a Swedish neurosurgical pioneer, Lars Leksell. Dr. Leksell was born in 1907 in Sweden. He graduated from the Karolinska school of medicine in 1935. He became a pioneer in the new field of stereotactic neurosurgery (see chapter 14) and invented a very popular stereotactic apparatus, the Leksell frame. In 1960, he succeeded his boss, Herbert Olivecrona, as professor and chair of neurosurgery at the Karolinska Institute.

As a young neurosurgical trainee, Leksell was dismayed by the frequent poor results of open neurosurgery. "The school of Olivecrona was hard. The trade could not be done better in any other place, but sometimes even his mastership did not suffice. Progress goes over heaps of corpses," said the great surgeon von Mikulicz. "But it was difficult to accept the high mortality and the failures fastened in my mind."

All neurosurgeons carry the burden of bad outcomes. These inevitable occurrences lead to many sleepless nights and to self-doubt. I believe each patient tragedy takes a little piece of your soul. Leksell is said to have described this feeling in the following story:

The little Jewish boy from Warsaw had bilateral acoustic neuromas. He lay on his face with his head on the ring-formed headrest. I was busy administering the anesthetic, sitting on the floor in the operation room. "Coagulation! Suck! Suck!" It seemed the bleeding could not be stopped. The boy started to breath more and more superficially and then stopped breathing altogether. After changing I went through the park and saw the father, the rabbi with the caftan, the round hat, the sidelocks, walking up and down, pale and restless, waiting for the outcome. I greeted him but did not dare to go and tell him what had happened.

Leksell wanted a better way. In 1951, he and a physicist, Börje Larsson, developed the radiosurgical concept and coined the term. Eventually they developed a radiosurgical device that they called the gamma knife. Multiple versions of the gamma knife have subsequently been installed in hundreds of institutions around the world. The gamma knife uses several hundred radioactive cobalt sources. Each source is focused on the target within the patient's brain. Since each radiation path goes through a different path to the brain, the normal brain gets very little radiation. But at the target, where all of the beams come together, a very concentrated dose of radiation is deposited. This outpatient technique has proven very effective at treating a number of brain lesions, including benign and some malignant brain tumors. A unit specifically designed for brain tumors was installed at the Karolinska in 1974. The first United States unit was installed in Pittsburgh in 1987. So, in 1985 we were very early into the radiosurgery game.

Radiosurgery is done by a team, including neurosurgeons, radiation oncologists, and radiation physicists. So, Al Rhoton and I made an appointment to meet with the chair of radiation oncology, Rod Million, and his chief of physics (whom I had never met), Frank Bova. Dr. Rhoton was a stickler for suit-and-tie dress at work. For some reason, on the day of the meeting, I didn't wear a tie. Dr. Rhoton let me know that he was embarrassed to be going to this meeting with me so dressed. We walked into Dr. Million's office. I was quietly amused to see Dr. Million dressed in jeans and a Guy Harvey fishing shirt! We agreed that we should expedite the development of a radiosurgical capability at the University of Florida.

Shortly thereafter, in January 1986, Frank and I flew with a young hospital administrator, Jodi Mansfield, to

Stockholm, Sweden. Stockholm is quite cold and dark in January. There, we were graciously received by the Elekta company (they manufactured the gamma knife) and by the neurosurgeons at the Karolinska. One day we watched radiosurgical pioneer Ladislau Steiner move from room to room on the neurosurgical ward, speaking four different languages to four different patients from other areas of Europe. That day he treated one young woman with an arteriovenous malformation. Back then, the treatment was done under general anesthesia. There was no computer planning. The treatment took most of the day.

The next day we traveled to Uppsala, where we met with Leksell's original collaborator, physicist Börje Larsson. We also visited the factory where the gamma knife was manufactured in Motala. At dinner on our last night we were saddened to learn that Lars Leksell, the founder of this feast, had just died while on vacation in Switzerland.

Back in Gainesville, we went to the Shands Hospital Board and persuaded them to buy what would have been the second gamma knife in the US. But Frank had substantial concerns about the gamma knife: it was very expensive, it could only be used on cranial lesions, the computer planning was very crude, and most importantly, the radioactivity of the cobalt sources decreased by half every five years, so the units would need to be reloaded. No one had actually ever done that. So, we began to consider alternatives that would use the linear accelerator (LINAC) as the source of radiation instead of cobalt sources. LINACs were then in common use for conventional radiation treatment of cancer. Their radiation output was essentially similar to that of a cobalt source, but they were not, at that time, accurate enough to focus hundreds of beams on a target.

In the 1980s, a number of LINAC radiosurgery pioneers, including Betti, Colombo, and Hartmann, published very early descriptions of their systems. In the US, Ken Winston, a neurosurgeon, and Wendell Lutz, a physicist, had a system operating at one of the Harvard hospitals. We flew to Boston and spent all day and part of the night watching them treat one patient. Frank and I came back convinced that we could correct the inadequacies of the existing LINAC systems and develop something better (like Leksell). We went back to the hospital and told them that if they funded us, we could develop a LINAC system that would be just as good as the gamma knife for one-quarter of the price.

Frank's idea for correcting the inaccuracies involved creating an add-on device in the Shands machine shop that would control the rotation of the accelerator and the rotation of the patient. He also saw a way to greatly improve the speed of the computer planning that was currently available. Frank began building the device. We hired Russell Moore, a talented young computer programmer, who began work on the dose planning system.

When the device was ready, we needed to install and test it on an actual linear accelerator. There was no time available on the single machine at Shands. But we were allowed to work on a LINAC at a satellite facility across town. It was available for research when all patient treatments were finished, usually around 5 p.m. Thus Frank and I began spending two to three evenings a week installing, testing, and refining our new LINAC radiosurgery machine. In April 1988, it was finally ready to go. We treated our first patient on May 10, 1988. The University of Florida patented the system, which was subsequently licensed to Philips, then Medtronic, then Varian, and installed in hundreds of hospitals around the world.

I proudly submitted a paper describing our work to the *Journal of Neurosurgery*. It was rejected because "it had no relevance to the field of neurosurgery." In 1989, the paper was published in *Surgical Neurology*. Similar to the evoked potential experience and the stereotactic surgery experience, as we published more and more papers describing our favorable results, invitations to speak at national and international meetings came in. But the reception was different this time. Evoked potentials did not threaten any existing neurosurgical procedures. They simply made them safer. Radiosurgery, however, was a disruptive technology.

As we and many other groups began to present mounting evidence that radiosurgery was at least as effective and much, much safer than conventional neurosurgery for many patient conditions, the neurosurgical establishment fought back. After all, we neurosurgeons had subjected ourselves to those brutal residencies and fellowships to learn how to do very complicated procedures. So, they must be better than some new paradigm shift, right?

For at least a decade, my presentations elicited responses like, "If you were a decent surgeon, you wouldn't need radiosurgery." Well, I was a decent surgeon. Then and now,

I was the go-to guy for the most difficult cases at UF. But shouldn't we always pick the procedure that is best for the patient? My story was that I did both things, so I had no ax to grind. I also reminded my audiences that, "If your only tool is a hammer, everything looks like a nail."

Today, four thousand nine hundred patients, one hundred fifty peer-reviewed papers, and hundreds of talks later, it's hard to find a hospital in the US without radiosurgical capability. It is absolutely mainstream. Of course, success in neurosurgery involves technical skill and mental toughness. But I am totally convinced that the ability to think outside the box, to ask "why are we doing it that way?", is also crucial to the advance of the field.

CURING THE INCURABLE | 16

I n early September 2001, I took Ransom and two of our three children to Australia for two medical meetings. The first meeting involved a group founded by Al Rhoton, called the International Society for Neurosurgical Instrument Inventors. It was to be held in Cairns, on the coast of northern Australia. The second meeting was much bigger. It was the biannual meeting of the World Congress of Neurological Surgery, to be held in Sydney. I had several talks to give at each meeting.

On September 10, we arrived at our comfortable hotel in Cairns, exhausted after about twenty-four hours of travel. The four of us ate dinner and went to bed. The next morning, my wife flipped on the TV, and we watched the second of two hijacked jets fly into the World Trade Center in New York. My family and I were halfway around the world on 9/11! As you may remember, all air traffic everywhere in the world was grounded for several days. So, we just went on with the meeting, although all of us from the United States were filled with worry and wanted to get home. On September 13, air travel resumed (only domestic), and we flew to Sydney for the second meeting. We checked into a truly beautiful apartment on Sydney Harbor, not realizing that much worse news awaited.

A message was waiting from John Tew. John was chair of neurosurgery at the University of Cincinnati. He and I were colleagues and friends. He had graciously served as honored guest when I was president of the Congress of Neurological Surgeons in 1998. John told me that my mother had a brain tumor and that it probably was a glioblastoma. Now the tables were turned, weren't they? I wasn't the concerned surgeon for an anxious patient and family. I was the concerned family. Frankly, I couldn't believe it. My mom was seventy-one and, heretofore, had been in perfect health. She was intelligent, hardworking, deeply compassionate, and very active mentally and physically. My wife and my kids loved her every bit as much as I did. My mother's mother had lived well into her nineties. I had hoped to have my mom as my trusted friend for many more years.

It was a few more days before international travel resumed. We took a nearly empty flight from Sydney to Los Angeles. Ransom and the kids flew home. I flew to Cincinnati. My sister and my father picked me up at the airport. My father seemed to have difficulty navigating the parking garage, but we made it home. My mom was in her nightgown. She was glad to see me, but she was also clearly scared. She had mild speech difficulty but was otherwise well. She had been having trouble writing and had been trying to contact me by email but couldn't type out the message.

The next day we met with Dr. Tew and went through the pre-op process. Part of the tumor lit up on MRI scan and was relatively superficial. Additional tumor did not enhance but extended all the way into a deep part of brain called the thalamus. We agreed that a gross total resection would not be possible but that Dr. Tew would remove as much as he could safely. Then I remembered two things: First, Mom had complained several years ago of intermittent tingling of her right hand. She underwent a workup for median nerve wrist entrapment (called carpal tunnel syndrome) that was negative. Second, a year before, after playing tennis at my house in Gainesville, she had a fainting spell and hit the floor hard. We took her to the ER for a few stitches. She was completely normal on exam, and an ECG showed minor cardiac issues, so we did not opt for a CT scan. In retrospect, the hand tingling was probably from the tumor, and the fainting spell was probably a seizure, also from the tumor. My mom probably had a lower-grade glioma for some time, which then transformed into a glioblastoma.

Surgery went very well. We took her home two days later in excellent condition. The house was the one I grew up in. It was uncharacteristically littered with boxes, because my parents had just sold it in preparation for a full-time move to their condominium in Marco Island, Florida. I asked Dad to try to get out of the sale and stay in Cincinnati. I told him that they were going to need all of their support structure over the next months. I tried as hard as I could to tell him that this was a deadly disease, but he wasn't having it, and I simply couldn't push it.

Several weeks later they arrived in Gainesville, where we had decided Mom would get her radiation treatment while staying with us. My colleague and friend, John Buatti, was using a slightly different treatment approach, involving twice-daily treatments over four weeks, so we opted for that. It was only after a meeting with another colleague and friend, Bill Mendenhall, that I think my parents finally understood the facts about glioblastoma survival. They stayed in Gainesville a few more weeks to participate in my youngest son's bar mitzvah. As per usual, my mother prepared and delivered a beautiful speech during the ceremony. My extended family all came to Gainesville for David (my son) and my mom. And off my parents went to their condo.

For a very brief time, things went well. We had a great dinner celebration for Mom's birthday on December 4. By the new year, however, she was having speech problems and left-sided weakness. Back to Gainesville for an MRI, which showed progression of that nonenhancing deeper part of the tumor. Out of desperation, we treated the recurrent tumor with radiosurgery. But the disease's progression was now relentless. My mom was left-handed, so I had hoped that this left-sided tumor might spare her speech. But it was not to be. Soon she could barely communicate and was paralyzed on the right side.

Now the support structure came to her. My two sisters, Susan and Amy, took turns coming to Marco Island to help with her care. Dad also hired twenty-four-hour-a-day nurses. We had a nice celebration of Passover in March, which Mom enjoyed. On July 1, 2002, she died.

As we gathered at her grave site in Cincinnati, I think I truly understood, for the first time, the full depth of anguish that this disease brings to its victims and all who love them.

So, what to do? Viktor Frankl was a young, brilliant, Viennese psychiatrist when he and his wife were sent to Auschwitz. He never saw his twenty-four-year-old wife again, for she perished there. He himself barely survived. He lived to write about his experiences in the concentration camp. He founded a new school of psychotherapy, called logotherapy, based on his conviction that man's most profound driving force is to find meaning.

One day, exhausted, frozen, and hungry, on a work detail far from the camp, Frankl's companion mentioned his wife. Frankl later wrote:

> That brought thoughts of my own wife to mind. And as we stumbled on for miles, slipping on icy spots, supporting each other time and again, dragging one another up and onward, nothing was said, but we both knew: each of us was thinking of his wife. Occasionally I looked at the sky, where the stars were fading and the pink light of the morning was beginning to spread behind a dark bank of clouds. But my mind clung to my wife's image, imagining it with an uncanny acuteness. I heard her answering me, saw her smile, her frank and encouraging look. Real or not, her look was then more luminous than the sun which was beginning to rise.

A thought transfixed me: for the first time in my

life I saw the truth as it is set into song by so many poets, proclaimed as the final wisdom by so many thinkers. The truth—that love is the ultimate and highest goal to which man can aspire. Then I grasped the meaning of the greatest secret that human poetry and human thought and belief have to impart: the salvation of man is through love and in love. I understood how a man who has nothing left in this world still may know bliss, be it only for a brief moment, in the contemplation of his beloved. In a position of utter desolation, when man cannot express himself in positive action, when his only achievement may consist in enduring his sufferings in the right way—an honorable way—in such a position man can, through loving contemplation of the image he carries of his beloved, achieve fulfillment. For the first time in my life I was able to understand the meaning of the words, "The angels are lost in perpetual contemplation of an infinite glory" (Frankl, 2006).

Frankl, in analyzing how he and others found the strength to survive Auschwitz, wrote further:

What was really needed was a fundamental change in our attitude toward life. We had to learn ourselves and, furthermore, we had to teach the despairing men, that it did not really matter what we expected from life, but rather what life expected from us. We needed to stop asking about the meaning of life, and instead to think of ourselves as those who were being questioned by life, daily and hourly. Our answer must consist not in talk and meditation, but in right action and in right conduct. Life ultimately means taking the responsibility to find the right answer to its problems and to fulfill the tasks which it constantly sets for each individual.

We can discover the meaning of life in three different ways: (1) by creating a work or doing a deed; (2) by experiencing something or encountering someone; and (3) by the attitude we take toward unavoidable suffering (Frankl, 2006).

In my search to find meaning in my mother's tragedy and in the tragedies of so many brain tumor patients just like her, I have devoted myself to transforming the University of Florida Department of Neurosurgery into a world-leading center for brain tumor treatment. As discussed above, we know very well that great surgery, great radiation therapy, and available chemotherapy will not provide a satisfactory answer. What is needed is a completely different approach. To that end, I began work on the Phyllis K. Friedman Professorship. A professorship is a fund that provides financial support to the occupant of that chair. After several years, friends, family, and a grateful patient had contributed over $1 million. But much, much more was needed.

I approached the Preston A. Wells foundation. The Wells foundation had been generous philanthropic contributors to UF Neurosurgery since I first met them in 1983. Now they stepped forward and donated $5 million toward establishing a funded brain tumor center. In 2011, they contributed a further $10 million. This was matched by $10 million from the University of Florida. With $25 million in funds, we set about recruiting one of the world's best brain tumor science teams. We found that team working at Duke University.

Duane Mitchell, MD, PhD, and eight of his friends migrated to UF in 2013. Since then we have recruited over one hundred faculty and staff whose work is solely focused on finding cures for malignant brain tumors. The focus has been immunotherapy, using the body's own immune system to find and kill cancer cells. One immunotherapy approach takes tumor cells harvested at the time of surgery and uses them to create a vaccine that is injected into the patient. Another approach takes the patient's own T cells (immunity cells) and sensitizes them to the tumor cells. Then they are injected back into the patient. We currently have six first-in-human immunotherapy protocols for adults and children with malignant tumors. It's early days, but we have seen some very promising responses.

Subsequently, the Wells Foundation has contributed yet another $10 million. Harris Rosen, a hotelier and philanthropist from Orlando, Florida, has contributed $12 million in memory of his young son, Adam, who died from a malignant brain tumor. Duane and his colleagues have brought in additional millions of dollars of NIH and foundation grants.

UF Health Neurosurgery is and will remain relentless in our determination to make a real difference for patients with malignant brain tumors. We seek to find our "meaning" by "creating a work or doing a deed" and "by the attitude we take toward unavoidable suffering."

HOW WE LEARN | 17

E very year, UF Health Neurosurgery interviews about
fifty top-notch senior medical students from around
the country who are interested in matching into
one of our three annual resident spots. One of their most
commonly repeated questions is, "What are you looking
for in a new neurosurgical resident?" I tell them that we
have a wide diversity of characteristics and talents amongst
our twenty-one largely successful residents. But they all
share three common traits: First, they are dedicated, lifelong students. Second, they have a degree of mental toughness, which is absolutely necessary to handle the eighty-hour
workweeks taking care of very sick patients, sometimes
with bad outcomes. Third, they are creative—they have the
ability to ask, "Why do we do it this way?" "Might there be
a better way?"

I cannot emphasize too highly the importance of being a
lifelong student. Virtually everything I do today in neurosurgery is different and, often, new, compared to what I did as
a brand-new faculty member in 1982. The phenomenal

growth in what we know and what we can accomplish in the clinical neurosciences is what makes the field so exciting and so rewarding. It's also sometimes what separates us academics from our very capable colleagues in private practice. At UF Health, I am constantly challenged by my colleagues and students to continuously improve and grow. To do so, I must be an avid reader/student, and I must be open to new ideas, new ways of doing things. This is a part of my job that I love.

As a dedicated, lifelong student and as a teacher of medical students, neurosurgery residents, and fellow neurosurgeons (through papers, talks, courses at national/international meetings), I have spent a lot of time thinking about how we learn.

Theory of knowledge is called epistemology in philosophical circles. Plato, who lived from 427–347 BC in Athens, established a philosophical school which he called the Academy. Plato's dialogues can be easily read today in a single large volume. Most of them are a series of conversations in which his teacher, Socrates, engages a large number of male characters. Plato was a dualist (see chapter 18). That is, he believed in the perceptual world we see around us and, also, in an intelligible but invisible world of "perfect forms." In the Meno, he addressed epistemology. In what is now known as Meno's paradox, Plato asked, "How can you learn something when you have no idea that what you don't know exists?" Today, we might say, usually about someone particularly ignorant, "He doesn't know what he doesn't know." Plato's answer doesn't satisfy today's readers. He said that learning was the discovery of preexisting knowledge—that the soul remembers those perfect forms from its previous life.

Aristotle, who lived from 384–322 BC in Athens, was Plato's student. His school was called the Lyceum. He invented logic, physics, zoology, botany, and coined the term metaphysics, which simply means after physics. He has been known ever since as "the Philosopher." Aristotle's works involve many, many volumes and can be challenging to digest. In terms of epistemology, his most enduring role was as the founder of syllogistic, deductive logic. This approach toward deriving the laws of the universe from simple observation and complex reasoning dominated Western thought through the Middle Ages.

In deductive reasoning, one starts with first principles, like Aristotle or the Bible, and derives all else logically. In every one of Aristotle's syllogisms there is a major and minor premise and a conclusion. For example: All mortal things die. All men are mortal things. Ergo, all men die. In Aristotle's system, there are 256 possible types of syllogisms. Only nineteen are logically valid, and they were all given a name. For example, syllogism one is called Barbara. Until the Renaissance, scholars routinely memorized all nineteen valid syllogisms and used them daily.

Fast-forward two thousand years to Francis Bacon, who lived in London from 1561–1626. He largely developed and popularized a different type of reasoning, called induction. Induction draws knowledge through observation, experimentation, and hypothesis testing—in other words, the modern scientific method. Many other philosophers have contributed much to the theory of knowledge, amongst them Berkeley, Hume, Kant, Wittgenstein, and Russell.

I have found three modern models of learning to be particularly informative: Dreyfus, Csikszentmihalyi, and Ericsson.

Brother philosophers Stuart and Hubert Dreyfus proposed a model of learning in 1980. In the Dreyfus model, students pass through six stages: novice, advanced beginner, competent, proficient, expert, and master (Dreyfus and Dreyfus, 1980). Novices are rule-followers. They are engaged in repeated practice, with supervision and feedback. In the real world this produces poor performance. They have no sense of the whole situation.

Examples: Shift gears when the tachometer reads four thousand RPMs. The knight moves two spaces up and one over. The surgical assistant should use suction to maintain a blood-free field.

The advanced beginner pays some attention to the overall situation. Appropriate coaching can improve his situational awareness. He follows maxims. The advanced beginner is nerve-wracked and exhausted by the multiple rules.

Examples: Upshift when the motor sounds like it is racing. Attack a weakened king's side. Listen to the sound of the suction to determine whether it is clogged.

The competent learner pays attention only to what's relevant and important. There aren't necessarily any rules to guide this process. If you fail, it's on you, it's not because someone didn't provide you with the rules. One needs to be emotionally involved in the outcome to reach this stage.

It is difficult because students don't want to hurt anyone, and they also don't want to look stupid.

Examples: Pay attention to car speed, surface conditions, criticality of time, etc. Don't pay attention to the loss of your own pieces if not critical to your chess attack. Select the appropriate suction size, verify function, adjust light, keep your head away from the light's path to the surgical site.

The proficient learner immediately sees the goals. He may not have enough experience to automatically know the answers and may still depend on some maxims and rules.

Examples: The proficient driver feels, in the seat of his pants, whether car speed is too great but must still choose a solution. The proficient chess player can recognize a large number of situations but still must choose amongst the responses. The proficient surgeon can feel how hard to pull on a tumor but still must consciously choose amongst movements.

An expert performs an action without thinking. There is no problem-solving involved. He has switched to a nonanalytic, nonplatonic, intuitive form of reasoning.

Examples: The chess grand master recognizes the board like a familiar face and knows the right sequence of moves without thinking. The expert neurosurgeon moves his hands hundreds of times without thinking and quickly and efficiently removes the tumor.

Finally, the master understands what it means to be a (you name it). He is never satisfied with his current level of knowledge. He understands the broad context and knows what is at stake. He doesn't follow rules, he breaks them.

I think the Dreyfus description of learning accurately portrays neurosurgical residency. It is now a seven-year program. Our first-year residents are novices. In the second and third year, they are frequently advanced beginners. In their fourth and fifth years (senior residency), they progress to competence. Most achieve proficiency, at least in the more common procedures, in the sixth and seventh years. In my estimation, it takes about ten years after that to approach mastery, usually in a much more narrow subspecialty area where you have had a lot of practice.

Profound objections to this model have recently emerged, as we better understand the fast and slow thinking mechanisms of the brain (see chapter 25).

In the 1980s, psychologist Mihaly Csikszentmihalyi coined the term "flow" (Csikszentmihalyi, 1990). Also known as "being in the zone," it's an experience that has seven key characteristics: First, one must be completely involved, focused, and concentrated either due to innate curiosity or training. Second, there is a sense of ecstasy, that is, being outside everyday reality. Third, there is great inner clarity—knowing what needs to be done and how well it is going. Fourth, one knows the activity is doable, that one's skills are adequate to the task, so one is neither anxious nor bored. Fifth, there is a sense of serenity. Sixth, one is so focused on the present that the passage of time isn't noticed. Seventh, whatever produces this "flow" feeling becomes its own reward.

If one constructs a graph with difficulty on the y-axis and ability on the x-axis, flow is achieved when ability precisely matches the challenge (when x equals the y). If the challenge is too great, one is anxious. If the challenge is too little, one is bored. Our residents spend a great deal of time in the anxious, advanced beginner zone taking care of problems they haven't seen before with the help of senior residents and faculty. As they approach the end of training for common, simple procedures, they may experience flow or even boredom. As they accumulate years of practice and approach mastery, they will require greater and greater challenges to achieve flow, spending more and more time in the boredom zone.

I frequently experience that flow feeling when I am taking out a challenging skull base tumor. I have also felt it as a runner—once I hit a certain pace and rhythm, I don't think about putting one foot in front of another. Time slows down and my thoughts clarify. I have also noticed it while skiing (although, not being an expert, I can also find myself in the anxiety zone). I have felt a flow feeling when delivering a talk particularly well to a large audience and I think this drives a lot of my colleagues in academic neurosurgery. I have felt it while shooting an instrument approach to the runway through the clouds in my airplane. I have never experienced a flow feeling while attending a committee meeting! I am sure everyone reading this book knows the flow feeling.

K. Anders Ericsson, professor of psychology at Florida State University, along with his colleagues, has popularized the concept of deliberate practice. According to Ericsson,

People believe that because expert performance is qualitatively different from a normal performance, the expert performer must be endowed with characteristics qualitatively different from those of normal adults. Only a few differences, most notably height, are genetically prescribed. Instead we argue that the differences between expert performers and normal adults reflect a life-long period of deliberate effort to improve performance in a specific domain (Ericsson and Kintsch, 1995).

Deliberate practice is more than just repeating a task. It involves expert feedback and continually practicing a skill at more challenging levels with the intention of achieving mastery. Others have stated that ten thousand hours of deliberate practice will lead to mastery in almost any field. Does it apply to neurosurgical training? Our residents spend most of their seven years with us working more than sixty hours per week. Let's make the gross assumption that this equates to ten hours of deliberate surgical practice per week (practice with expert assistance, where the resident is the principle surgeon) for forty-five weeks a year. That's four hundred and fifty hours per year. That means that one would become expert in at least some areas of neurosurgery twenty-two years after starting training. This seems about right to me in terms of achieving "mastery" in the neurosurgical operating room. I think it's undeniable that the more supervised time our residents get in the operating room, the quicker they will achieve competence and, ultimately, mastery.

THE MIND | 18

*What a piece of work is man, how noble in reason, how
infinite in faculties, in form and moving how express and
admirable, in action how like an angel, in apprehension
how like a god! The beauty of the world, the paragon of
animals. And yet, to me, what is this quintessence of dust?*
—Hamlet, Shakespeare

istorically, all of science was once the purview of
philosophy. As systematic approaches were developed in each of many fields like astronomy, mathematics, and physics, they peeled off from philosophy and
became separate sciences. For some fields, the easier parts
are now science, while the many unanswered questions
remain in the philosophical domain. That's where we
stand today with our understanding of how the brain creates the mind.

In the seventeenth century, René Descartes explained
what we can call "the mind-brain problem" by creating a
dualistic explanation of the universe, called substance
dualism. This theory holds that there are two kinds of substances in the world, mental and physical. The essence of
the mental is consciousness. The essence of the physical is
dimensions. Minds are indivisible and indestructible.

Minds are known directly, while bodies are known indirectly. The mental is the realm of religion and the physical, the realm of science.

But there are many problems with substance dualism: In a dualistic universe, how can the mind and body interact? How can I know other people have minds since I only have access to my own mind? How can people sleep if a person consists of mind, and the mind is essentially conscious? And many more. Various attempts to solve these problems have usually failed. The failure to solve dualism's problems has led to the widespread acceptance of monism, the view that there is only one type of substance. One type of monism, called materialism, is the view that only matter exists. That has become the dominant view today in both science and philosophy. Modern philosophy of mind is largely an attempt to get a version of materialism that is not subject to decisive objections.

One branch of materialism, called the strong artificial intelligence (AI) theory, posits that the brain is like a computer, only much, much more powerful. Indeed, there is no computer in existence today that can match the massive parallel-processing capability of the brain. But many futurists suggest that it is just a matter of time before new kinds of computers will reach and exceed the processing power of the human brain. When that happens, Kurzweil says, we will have reached a singularity when computers become conscious. Alan Turing, one of the founders of modern computing, developed a simple test, since called the Turing test. If an expert cannot distinguish the behavior of a computer or a human behind a screen, then the machine must have the same cognitive abilities as the human, including consciousness.

The strong AI hypothesis is very popular. But there are several strong philosophical objections. One is called Searle's Chinese Room argument. Imagine that a monolingual English speaker is locked in a room with a set of rules for answering questions in Chinese. As each Chinese question comes through a window, the English speaker goes to an enormous book of rules and finds the Chinese answer, which he passes out of the room. The English speaker has answered the question without knowing a word of Chinese!

Searle argues that this is how a computer works. It has an enormous capacity to follow its rules (the program) but has no understanding or consciousness. "Programs are syntactical, minds have semantic contents, syntax is not sufficient for semantics therefore programs are not minds" (Searle, 1980). He argues further that we simply do not know how something semantic arises from something non-semantic, although it clearly happens all the time in the brain.

Chalmers says that we have made great progress in solving "the easy problems." We know a lot about the brain's ability to discriminate, categorize, and react to stimuli. We also know much about how a cognitive system integrates information, how it accesses its inner states, how it reports on its own mental states, and how it can focus attention and behavior. But there is an explanatory gap between the dynamics of the nervous system and the nature of consciousness. Qualia (i.e., redness, taste, pain, grief, love, etc.) are not in any way now known reducible to neural events (Chalmers, 1996).

And so, today, we are stuck with the "hard problem of consciousness." Consider Thomas Nagel's article, "What Is It Like to Be a Bat?" He argues that an organism has a conscious mental state only if there is something that it is to be that organism. How does echolocation "feel"? What is it like for a bat to be a bat?

Or try Frank Jackson's article, "What Mary Knew" (Jackson, 1986). Mary is a neuroscientist who knows everything there is to know about the science of color, but she has lived her entire life in a black and white room. If she goes out into the real world, does she learn something new? If yes, then our science leaves out something about the experience of color, so physicalism must be wrong. And this brings us back to the concept of dualism. Physicalism appears to fail because thoughts are not like things, and feelings have no shape, leading many to feel that the physicalist agenda is overly optimistic. But others feel that this is premature, that we simply do not have the science that we need at this time. Penrose and others have concluded that the phenomenon of mental life may require a physical science not yet at hand.

In neuromedicine we are called upon, not infrequently, to help patients with the most severe loss of consciousness, which we call coma. Coma results from a wide variety of brain injuries including trauma, hemorrhage, stroke, infection, and others. Comatose patients don't open their eyes or respond to verbal stimuli. Even with a great deal of experience, it can be difficult to predict when and if a given comatose patient might awaken. Although very rare, some comatose patients have awakened after months or years in a noncommunicative state. Some of these patients have even complained about conversations they have overheard while comatose.

Mr. J was a middle-aged man with a two-year history of hearing loss in his left ear. He also had imbalance and facial numbness on the left. Evaluation revealed a large, left-sided vestibular schwannoma. Vestibular schwannomas are benign tumors that grow from the superior vestibular nerve. As they enlarge, the back part of the brain, including the cerebellum and brainstem, is compressed. For large tumors, surgery is the only option.

On the day of surgery, we transported the patient to the operating room. After the induction of anesthesia, we placed the patient in the right-side-down position. He was prepped and draped. We made an incision behind his left ear and removed a quarter-sized piece of bone. We opened the dura and drained spinal fluid to relax the cerebellum. We then draped the operating microscope. Using the microscope's magnification and lighting, we easily identified the tumor. Vestibular schwannomas are removed by entering the tumor, removing the inside of the tumor, and then carefully peeling the tumor capsule away from the normal brain structures. After three hours, the tumor was out. The patient awakened basically normal.

That afternoon I visited with him as he was up in a chair and talking with his family. Around midnight, he became somnolent. My resident phoned me, and we reviewed the CT scan. The tumor was gone, but the patient had developed hydrocephalus, or water on the brain, a known risk of brain tumor surgery. Per plan, the resident went ahead and placed a small drainage tube, through a small hole drilled in the skull, into the fluid cavity. The patient did not respond. A repeat CT scan revealed bleeding in the fluid cavity and along the drainage tube track. Another drain was placed, this time successfully, on the other side. Days, and then several weeks went by without substantial recovery. The patient was comatose. I was, as always, devastated by this unexpectedly poor turn of events.

I did not think the patient was going to make a meaningful recovery and discussed that multiple times with his wife. He had a living will—a document stating that he did not want to be sustained in a comatose state. She insisted that he would recover, given time. So off he went to a care center for comatose patients. Six weeks later, she and her husband walked into the clinic! He was substantially recovered and very happy to be alive. And I was very happy that his wife hadn't listened to me.

So, here is a hard problem for neurosurgeons: We have a duty not to exploit the vulnerabilities of others. Just how much biological function must a creature have to enjoy some measure of respect? On what criteria do those with a living will base their judgment of a life not worth living? And should we respect it? We don't know what it's like to be in a coma any more than we know what it's like to be a bat.

HEALTH-CARE REFORM | 19

Nobody ever went broke underestimating the
intelligence of the American public.
—H.L. Mencken

I n 1965, as part of Lyndon Johnson's war on poverty, and against great opposition from the American Medical Association, Congress passed the first Medicare/Medicaid laws. Medicare was designed to provide those age sixty-five and up greatly discounted medical care by essentially providing that group with universal federal health insurance. Part A has evolved to cover 80 percent of hospital expenses. Part B covers, to varying degrees, the physician bill. Medicaid was slightly different. It has now become a partnership between the states and the feds, providing health insurance for those falling below a percentage of the federal poverty line, the disabled, and several other groups (mainly children). At the time, the predominant model was fee-for-service. But there weren't a lot of expensive medical services (like most elective brain surgery today) available at that time. So, some paid cash. Insurance policies of the day, like Blue Cross/Blue Shield, typically reimbursed 80 percent of the "usual and customary fee." Those who couldn't pay and didn't have insurance didn't get much in the way of medical care.

By the time I got to medical school in 1973, Medicare/Medicaid was having a significant impact on our health-care system. A tremendous boom in hospital construction was underway. Physicians, now reimbursed at a high rate for their "usual and customary fees," at least in the Medicare and insured groups, were making increasingly high salaries. Likewise, a boom in medical technology was yielding ever-greater advances in imaging, surgical techniques, and medical approaches to diseases like cancer and heart disease that theretofore had very few treatment options. It was an exciting time to become a neurosurgeon because it was becoming safer, more effective, and more precise.

Flash forward to 2020. I am sixty-seven and have stepped down after twenty years as chair of UF Health Neurosurgery. It is clear that Lyndon Johnson's baby has grown up and become somewhat of a disgrace compared to most other national health-care programs. It's not a Medicare/Medicaid problem. But almost everything else has become perverted. Why? Because every incentive in our current system is misaligned. Patients who have insurance that covers their medical expenses have little incentive to be prudent in their use of services or, more importantly, to take better care of themselves. Under the continuing fee-for-service model, doctors and hospitals get paid more if they do more, so they do more, even when not indicated. Fear of medical malpractice suits has led to expensive defensive medicine. Insurance companies have hired hosts of medical directors whose job it is to deny requests to fund needed care. And worst of all, in the United States, drug and medical device manufacturers charge whatever they want, with virtually no price regulation.

Hence we have an enormous, inefficient, very expensive health-care system. We spend more than $8,000/person per year on medical care. That's twice what the next-highest country (Great Britain) spends. In 2010, the total tab was $2.6 trillion and accounted for 18 percent of the US Gross Domestic Product. As of 2017, the government was paying almost 50 percent of the total health-care expenses through Medicare and Medicaid. Because of politics during World War II, employees do not pay taxes on employer-provided health-care insurance, which results in a $200 billion tax shortfall. Most disgracefully, over eight hundred thousand Americans declare bankruptcy each year due to medical expenses!

But it's really much worse! 75 percent of our health-care costs are attributable to chronic disease, much of which is linked to smoking and obesity. The US has the highest rate of obesity in the world. And we are proud that we have gotten the smoking rate down to 24 percent! An astounding 30 percent of Medicare costs are spent in the last year of life on often futile care measures, frequently in a hospital intensive care unit. Nearly half of our population die in the hospital instead of at home. Insurance companies spend upwards of 30 percent of every health insurance premium dollar on administrative costs. These costs include reimbursement of stockholders, executives, and employees, all of whom contribute virtually nothing to actual health care. And across the country, there is a vast range of costs for the very same procedures. And even on the low end, those costs are usually higher than in any other county. Drug costs are much higher across the board in the US.

Well, you might say, that's expensive, but we really get the best health care in the world, right? Wrong! The US actually ranks last amongst the world's eleven wealthiest countries in health-care outcomes. You name it—infant mortality, cardiac event survival, stroke care, life expectancy, etc. We don't do as well as countries that spend a lot less money.

Fee-for-service is the health-care model from hell. It has led to a health-care constituency that fights every attempt to reduce expenses, because reducing health expenses means their own income will decrease. That includes physicians, hospitals, drug companies, insurance companies, and even patients. Let's review a bit more information on a few of these health-care hogs.

Physicians, through the AMA and many other lobbies, have fought every single attempt at health-care reform. Physician incomes, at least for specialists, are higher than any other country. Proceduralists, like me, make, by far, the most money. But, the real benefits in national health require the management of primary-care diseases like hypertension, diabetes, and obesity. Physicians have also been very resistant to following standardized guidelines— they simply don't want to be told what to do. And physicians as a group have done a very poor job of identifying and disciplining the small percentage who account for the majority of true malpractice. Physicians have teamed up with drug and device manufacturers to embark on a never-ending series of expensive but ultimately ineffective new procedures and treatments. In my own field, neurosurgery, I have witnessed suboccipital craniectomies for chronic fatigue, cerebellar stimulation for cerebral palsy, implanted radioactive isotopes for malignant brain tumors, laser spine surgeries—all of these procedures have either been disproven or are of marginal value, but thousands of patients have received them (and continue, in some cases, to receive them).

In the ten years between 1998 and 2008, the number of spinal fusions performed in the US doubled. Why? Sometimes it was because it was a relatively new procedure that could really help the patients. But as the number seen in 2018 continues to skyrocket, and as the number of fused patients with no improvement continue to jam my clinic, one suspects that the driver is the very high surgical fee associated with fusion.

That's not the worst of it. Several neurosurgeons whom I have helped train are in active collusion with accident attorneys to charge obscene fees for their procedures. Here's how it works: A patient sustains a spine injury in an auto or industrial accident. The patient hires an accident attorney. The attorney sends the patient to the neurosurgeon. The implicit understanding is that if the neurosurgeon certifies that the patient needs surgery, the attorney will reimburse the doctor directly from the legal proceeds for the surgical fee. So instead of getting $3,000 from Medicare for the procedure, the surgeon gets $100,000! This is an obscene perversion of our

Hippocratic oath and is a direct result of the fee-for-service system.

What about the hospitals? Their number is ever increasing. There are now over five thousand hospitals in the US, generating ever-increasing profit margins. And because of the fee-for-service system, every hospital wants every possible piece of the latest, expensive medical equipment. This ultimately means that many of these hospitals are performing low numbers of complex procedures. Low numbers of complex procedures, like coronary artery bypasses, carotid endarterectomies, and skull base tumor neurosurgeries, lead to relatively poor results. In other words, institutions that have providers who do high numbers of such procedures produce better results, usually at a lower cost. Community hospitals should stick to common medical problems and refer the rare complex problems to regional centers. Although this happens to some degree, frequently it doesn't. Hospitals, driven by fee-for-service, are loath to transfer patients. They are usually held responsible by their boards for the financial bottom line, not for patient outcomes.

As mentioned before, drug and device companies in the US charge as much as they possibly can, because insurance or federal programs will usually reimburse their price. Medicare, incredibly, is currently prohibited by law (the drug companies have a very large lobbying effort) from negotiating drug prices, as is done in almost every other country. So drug companies make their money in the US, while across the border in Canada, the same drug is much cheaper. In many instances, there is no proven difference in efficacy between an older generic drug and a new, more expensive drug. But the drug industry, through a multibillion-dollar marketing program directed to patients and physicians, has been remarkably effective in selling the more expensive options. When new drugs or devices provide an exciting breakthrough in medical care, they are frequently shockingly expensive. For example, it is nearly miraculous that Solvadi cures hepatitis C, but the cost of treatment is $84,000 (for pills!). Hep C treatment alone costs the health-care system $8 billion per year. Drug expenses are going up by about $50 billion per year!

So wasn't the Affordable Care Act (Obamacare) supposed to fix this mess? Obamacare is a three-legged program. The first leg is the mandate—almost every citizen and legal resident MUST have health insurance. The second leg involved subsidies; it replaced the state-by-state definitions of who qualified for Medicaid with one formula: Medicaid is to include everyone with income less than 133 percent of the federal poverty level. Medicaid expansion to cover these additional enrollees was to be funded largely by the federal government for the first five years, with lesser but still substantial subsidies thereafter. Insurance exchanges would provide insurance options and would provide individual subsidies to those with income up to less than 400 percent of the poverty level. The third leg required that insurance companies could not deny insurance to those with health issues. It also required companies to use at least 85 percent of the premium dollars on actual health care.

Please note that the system cannot work if any of the

legs are removed. Insurance companies cannot provide access to every patient, regardless of their health status, unless everyone, including the young, healthy population, is required to have insurance. Think about it. If young, healthy individuals could simply wait until they became ill to buy insurance, why in the world would they get it before? Eliminating the mandate simply drops most of the healthy patients out of the insured pool, leaving a sicker group, leading to higher premiums, leading to more people dropping out, etc. This is called the death spiral. Indeed, Congress has just done exactly that. They've kept the requirement that insurance not deny coverage, but they've eliminated the mandate. And insurance premiums are estimated to go up by 18 percent next year!

Unfortunately, even before it was hobbled by the Supreme Court and the current Congress, Obamacare failed to address many of the structural problems with our crazy fee-for-service system. It didn't change the way we paid for health care, it just added more insured people to a broken system. It didn't do much to control costs. Unintended consequences have included geographical consolidation of health-care systems to exert more leverage in contracting with insurance companies. New billion-dollar industries focused on quality improvement, and electronic medical records have emerged. And it's not clear that health care is actually better.

Other countries have taken a variety of approaches to generate health-care systems with better outcomes and lower prices. In the United Kingdom, taxes pay for everything. There are no bills for standard services. The government owns the hospitals and employs its workers. General practitioners act as gatekeepers. Patients have excellent access to primary care and emergency services, but there are long waits for specialty services like elective surgery.

In Japan, insurance pays for everything, but insurance companies are not allowed to make a profit. Most care is through private providers, and access is immediate. All fees are rigidly price-controlled. Our own Veterans Administration hospital system is like England. Medicare is a bit like Japan, but without the rigid price controls on everything.

The path forward requires a health-care system based on fairness and dignity for all. Coverage will be universal. Standard health care will be covered (not cosmetic surgery, for example). Medical and surgical care must be clearly supported by available evidence or, if evidence is not available, by consensus expert opinion.

It must control costs. That means insurance must go. The common employer-provided insurance system makes our businesses more expensive and less competitive. It makes it difficult for employees to leave a job they don't like for fear of losing insurance coverage. Health care, in the future, will be paid for via taxes. Just like Social Security and Medicare, these taxes will go into a trust fund. The trust fund will not be raided for other purposes. Each citizen will be given an annual health-care voucher that can be used to purchase health care from the regional integrated health-care organization of their choice. Each of these systems will be financially responsible for the total medical care of all individuals in that system. The fee-for-service model will end.

Systems will also, very importantly, be responsible for the quality of care provided. Routine care will be provided in many smaller locations. Complex care will concentrate volumes in fewer locations, producing better outcomes and lower costs. Patients will have ready access to the outcome data of all health-care organizations. Those systems that produce good results, including patient satisfaction, will prosper. Those that don't will fail. Yes, this will cost a lot of money in new taxes, but the total cost, that amazingly high percentage of GDP, will go down. That money could be used for many other national needs—infrastructure, education, national high-speed rail, green energy, etc.

The bottom line is that our health-care system must become totally patient-centric. Patients deserve the best possible care at an affordable cost. None of the constituencies that currently benefit from the fee-for-service system— doctors, insurance companies, drug companies, hospitals, and insured patients—will cooperate. It will take a crisis. The once-in-a-lifetime (we hope) COVID pandemic may be that crisis. As more than five million Americans have lost their employer-mandated health insurance (they are bankrupt), mustn't we think about a new approach?

ORLANDO | 20

No matter how cynical I get, it's never enough.
—Lily Tomlin

n 2012, UF Health leadership was approached by the
leadership of a similar-sized hospital in Orlando, called
the Orlando Regional Medical Center (ORMC). It was
the only Level I trauma center in a large metropolitan
area. They had struggled for more than a decade to recruit
and retain neurosurgeons, either in private practice in
Orlando or as hospital-employed physicians. Despite the
fact that they were paying the princely sum of $4,000/day
to take call, it turned out that it wasn't enough to convince
most neurosurgeons to stay up at night taking care of these
very ill patients.

ORMC approached Tim Flynn, our chief of staff, and
Tim Goldfarb, our hospital CEO, with a proposal for UF
Health Neurosurgery to take over neurosurgical services at
their hospital. I was opposed, seeing much hardship for my
department if we tried to pull this off. After all, Orlando
was more than one hundred miles away, and the culture of
their practice was thoroughly private practice, not academic. Nonetheless, off we went, along with Dick Lister,

my associate chair, and John Regenfuss, my departmental administrator and right-hand man.

On that first visit, we met the hospital administration. We toured the facility, which was large but rather worn. We met the neurosurgeons and neurologists currently on staff. We also visited their partner hospital, the Arnold Palmer Children's Medical Center. We actually met Arnold Palmer, who was there that day for a fundraiser. We went back home and came up with a proposal: UF Health would employ all of the neurosurgeons who were interested in joining us. We would set about hiring enough additional neurosurgeons to cover the trauma call. In the meantime, my faculty in Gainesville, if they wanted, would travel to Orlando to cover call, as needed.

We were determined that the neurosurgeons we employed would be topflight and would be fully integrated into the Gainesville department. They would have the same privileges and responsibilities, especially in the area of quality improvement. We agreed to pay them $100,000 per year above neurosurgeons with similar experience in Gainesville, as a community practice adjustment, mainly to do with the lack of resident support on call. ORMC would reimburse UF for all expenses and would pay my department a $500,000 per year management fee. This was subsequently raised to $750,000 per year.

Not surprisingly, a number of the ORMC physicians had significant concerns about UF coming to "their house." Only one neurosurgeon decided to accept our employment offer, German Montoya. German was seventy-nine years old. He had enjoyed a very distinguished record as an Orlando neurosurgeon for almost his entire career. He was very youthful and energetic. He was a good neurosurgeon and a wonderful gentleman. Another neurosurgeon agreed to take call but decided to remain in private practice. One of our seventh-year trainees, already board eligible (meaning he could take call and bill on his own), decided to spend his last training year in Orlando. So we had three people taking call. That meant that my colleagues and I needed to take the rest.

ORMC rapidly remodeled space and created an excellent office/clinic for us. I rented a condominium in downtown Orlando (at the Vue) and started spending every Saturday, Sunday, and Monday in Orlando, much of it on call. It felt strange to be on call by myself (no residents, no extenders), doing surgery in the middle of the night and rounding on dozens of patients every day. I also ran one day of clinic per week and started doing elective surgery in Orlando as well. In Gainesville, I had been off the call schedule since I turned sixty. When I had been on call, I always worked with a resident, which was often fun. In Orlando, alone, it wasn't fun, it was just work. Nonetheless, I felt I couldn't possibly convince my faculty to take call unless I did it myself. I also couldn't undertake the recruiting challenge and the practice transformation unless I led.

We rapidly succeeded in recruiting several more faculty. Josh Billingsley was one of our endovascular fellows. Jack Farkas was my age and was a veteran Florida private practice neurosurgeon. We also hired a neurologist who was endovascular-trained. Endovascular surgery involves treating neurosurgical issues like aneurysms or strokes by threading a catheter through the large artery in the leg (the femoral artery) and up to the brain blood vessels. For an acute stroke patient with an occluded brain vessel, emergent endovascular treatment can remove the clot and turn a devastating neurological future into no deficit at all. The addition of this expertise to the neurosurgical faculty in Orlando enabled ORMC to become a comprehensive stroke center. The hospital went from treating no strokes to dominating the Orlando market for these cases.

We hired a few more and lost a few, but at the end of four years we had five excellent, fellowship-trained UF neurosurgeons, living and working full time in Orlando. Bob Hirshl became our very capable associate chair for Orlando and was the local supervisor. I gave up my apartment after one year and started making day trips every Monday to run faculty meetings, help manage the practice, run a clinic, and participate in the quality program. Before we came, very few of the ORMC neurosurgeons had ever been to a quality improvement conference. Now it was a condition of employment. They became conversant with quality measures, implemented the same protocols we had developed in Gainesville, and saw dramatic improvements.

As promised, the Orlando faculty were fully implemented into our department. They came to Gainesville for departmental research weekend, graduation, and social events. We continued to go to Orlando to help with call. We had at least one combined tele-video pre-op conference every month. And everyone was pleased that Orlando became a favorite elective rotation for our trainees.

On June 12, 2016, I was on call in Orlando. Around 4 a.m., the emergency room attending called me and said they needed help right away. On that morning, Omar Mateen, a twenty-nine-year-old security guard, killed forty-nine people and wounded fifty-eight others inside the Pulse Nightclub. Pulse is two blocks from ORMC, so most of the forty-four injured people were transported to us. Nine of those patients ultimately died at ORMC.

Needless to say, I have never seen anything like what happened in the ORMC emergency room. I was struck by how well my colleagues in emergency medicine, trauma surgery, and intensive care rapidly organized, triaged the patients, and provided superb medical and surgical care. ORMC performed a total of seventy-six surgeries on these patients. More than a third of the deceased victims were shot in the head. None of those with head wounds survived to make it to the ER. One patient had a devastating abdominal injury. He survived emergency surgery but had a permanent spinal cord injury, causing paraplegia. There wasn't much for a neurosurgeon to do but watch in amazement.

After rounds that afternoon, I walked the two blocks back to the hotel where I was staying while on call. The hotel had become the family emergency center for food, water, medical care, and most importantly, updates on how the victims were doing. I watched as ORMC administration, along with Orlando police, announced the names of the dead. I have never in my life seen so much abject grief, misery, and wailing. It seemed like a scene from Dante's *Inferno.* I will never forget the screaming as long as I live.

At our monthly medical leadership executive committee meeting, I filled in the group on my observations that night. I told them that we should be very proud to be part of a group of physicians, nurses, and staff that had performed so admirably in the face of extreme adversity.

About six months later, I received a registered letter from the CEO of ORMC, informing me that UF Health services would no longer be needed. There was no forewarning, no meeting, no face-to-face conversations, no recognition of the blood sweat, toil, and tears we had willingly invested in their organization. We had succeeded so well in building a high-quality neurosurgical service that it wished to dissolve its association with UF. The five neurosurgeons we had hired didn't want to leave UF. But they all had family, friends, houses, etc. in Orlando. In return for a buyout fee, we released them all from their noncompete agreements, and they became ORMC employees. As far as I know they are all doing well.

One of the things that most bothers physicians these days is that hospital/med school administrations often seem to treat them as replaceable cogs. There is a saying that "we may love the organization, but the organization doesn't love us back." That's certainly been my experience at UF Health, where I've spent my entire career and, obviously, at ORMC. That's okay, the rewards of caring for patients with neurosurgical problems are so incredibly great that this organizational disrespect pales in significance. As I often tell my colleagues and trainees, "Thank God the neurosurgery is so easy, because the rest of it will drive you crazy."

ROBERT WATSON | 21

Academic politics are so brutal because the stakes are so small.
—Henry Kissinger

first met Robert Watson when I was a neurosurgery resident. I spent three months on Neurology, one with the chairman, Mel Greer, one with a chairman-to-be, Ed Valenstein, and one with Bob Watson. The month with Watson was remarkable as Bob was a very, very good teacher. Even today, I have my notes from his lectures on dementia, neurological emergencies, etc. On rounds, he was a remarkable bedside diagnostician. The ability of an astute clinician to localize and diagnose from a really good neurological history and physical had attracted me to neurosurgery to start with. I loved my neurology rotation, especially my month with Bob. He became a valued teacher and mentor.

Bob was twelve years older than me. He had grown up in Nashville, Tennessee. His family then moved to Tampa. He attended the University of Florida as an undergrad and a medical student. He also did his neurology residency at UF. After a short period on faculty, he went into private practice in Pensacola. But he really missed the teaching, so he returned to UF and quickly rose through the ranks to become a professor of neurology. He is the best bedside neurologist and the best teacher I have ever met.

I crossed paths with Bob many more times during residency and early faculty days. When I was chief resident at the VA Hospital, he called to consult on a patient, Colonel H. The colonel was eighty and was admitted to Neurology for evaluation of progressive dementia, incontinence, and gait difficulty. The gait problem was now so bad that he was basically curled up in bed most of the time. The diagnosis was normal pressure hydrocephalus (NPH). NPH is a condition where the fluid cavities of the brain enlarge even though the spinal fluid pressure is normal. The cause is usually unknown. The resulting pressure on the frontal lobes and the descending pathways from the frontal lobes to the brainstem causes the classic triad of symptoms: dementia, incontinence, and gait disturbance. The treatment involves the surgical insertion of a tube into the brain-fluid cavity. The tube is then tunneled through a series of small skin incisions to the abdomen, where it is inserted into the peritoneal cavity. The fluid that is blocked up in the head drains through the tube and is reabsorbed in the abdomen.

Several days after surgery, I saw Colonel H with Bob Watson. He was not only ambulatory, but he was so happy that he actually danced a jig in front of us! What a great outcome! I saw Colonel H back in clinic two weeks later for suture removal. His wife said, "The colonel is a wonderful lover. Is it safe for him to have sex?" An even better outcome!

Neurology and Neurosurgery met once a month at 7 a.m. for a clinicopathological conference (CPC), wherein a puzzling case was presented by neuropathology. The possible diagnoses were presented. Then, usually, the results of an autopsy, including a detailed analysis of the brain, were presented. On one particular Friday morning, a case was presented where, after multiple swings in sodium levels, a patient developed findings of brainstem dysfunction, then became comatose and died. The case was discussed by Steve Nadeau, a young Neurology faculty member. He settled on a diagnosis of fungal meningitis. Other opinions were solicited.

I raised my hand and named a rare disorder called central pontine myelinolysis. That turned out to be correct!

When I got back to my office, the phone rang. It was Bob Watson. "Congratulations, you sumbitch!" By an outstanding coincidence, some years later, I was a visiting faculty at New York Medical College. At their grand rounds, they presented a case of "tomaculous neuropathy," a rare peripheral nerve disease. Some months later, in Gainesville, guess what? The CPC case was tomaculous neuropathy, which I was able to nail. I think these and other shared cases and conferences convinced Bob that I was a serious student of neurology, and our friendship continued to grow.

Around the time that I became chair of UF Neurosurgery, I discovered that Bob and I shared a deep interest in Civil War history. He was going to a meeting in Washington, DC. I flew up and picked him up on the last day of the meeting. We drove to Gettysburg. We spent a great two days there. Then off we went to Antietam and Harper's Ferry. We took another self-guided trip to Richmond, Petersburg, and Appomattox. Then we began taking guided group trips. Over the years we have been to Shiloh, Fredericksburg, Manassas, and Chancellorsville. We have studied Sherman's march from Chattanooga to Atlanta. We have followed the trail of John Wilkes Booth from Ford's Theatre to his fatal capture in Virginia. We have done the Overland campaign, encompassing the Battle of the Wilderness, Spotsylvania Courthouse, the North Anna, and Cold Harbor. We've been to Vicksburg and have studied Lee's retreat from Petersburg to Appomattox. In short, we've spent a LOT of time together learning about the Civil War and having a lot of fun.

Our favorite tour guide is Ed Bearss. He is now ninety-seven years old and no longer vigorous. Ed grew up in rural Montana. After Pearl Harbor, he enlisted in the Marines and fought in the Pacific theater. He was severely wounded and lost the use of most of his left arm. After prolonged hospitalization and recovery stateside, he went to college and went to work for the National Park Service. He rose to the position of chief historian of the Park Service. He is widely recognized as the greatest living Civil War battlefield guide. Bob and I invited Ed to UF years ago. He spoke to our med students about Civil War medicine, and we visited local Civil War–era graveyards. Ed seems to know just about everything there is to know about the war in incredible detail. His tours are incredibly informative and very entertaining,

Bob spent his last seventeen years at UF doing

neurology part-time and serving as the senior associate dean for students full time. He and his colleague, Lynn Romrell, did much to improve the quality of the UF medical students. They were known nationally for their excellence. The senior associate dean is also in charge of resident education. The governing body for all residencies in the US is the ACGME (the Accreditation Council for Graduate Medical Education). The ACGME had decided that each institution sponsoring residencies must have an Institutional Graduate Medical Education Committee (ICGME). The ICGME would ensure that each of the many residencies met all of the general requirements. And presiding over the ICGME would be the Designated Institutional Official (DIO).

I was the residency program director for neurosurgery, and Bob asked me to organize UF's first ICGME and to become the DIO. We both dived into the arduous process of setting up the committee and ensuring institutional compliance with the ACGME's many new rules. We nervously went through the ACGME site visit and passed with flying colors.

About twelve years ago, a new dean, Dr. Bruce Kone, got sideways with Watson. Bob had taken the standard UF state retirement option five years earlier. It's called DROP and basically allows UF faculty to receive some retirement benefits early. When the retirement date came, it was standard operating procedure for those faculty to be rehired if they wished so. During his tenure as associate dean, Bob had raised millions of dollars from the Chapman Foundation to establish the Chapman Humanism Center for UF med students. This center actively promoted and educated medical students on the vitally important humanistic aspects of medical care. Bob planned to continue with educational duties and to remain in the endowed chair established by the Chapmans. Dr. Kone offered to rehire him, but only if Bob would work as a full-time neurologist, something he hadn't done for seventeen years.

Bob objected. On the Wednesday before Thanksgiving, Dr. Kone sent an email to all of the clinical chairs, myself included. It was a mean-spirited, insulting diatribe, enumerating his reasons for not rehiring Bob. I called Dr. Kone and told him that he could say anything he wished to faculty behind closed doors, but that this kind of email character assassination was unheard of. About thirty minutes later, I sent an email to Dr. Kone and all of the clinical chairs. In it, I reviewed Bob's years of superb service as a great clinician and associate dean. I suggested that any reasonable boss would treat him with the greatest of dignity and courtesy. And I directly refuted many of Dr. Kone's allegations. Then off I went to have Thanksgiving with my family.

On Friday, Dr. Kone called me and told me to be in his office at 6 a.m. on Monday. I was there at six. He didn't show until 6:45. Once again, he renewed his criticisms of Bob. I told him I thought I had made it clear that Bob was my friend and that I wasn't interested in his scurrilous comments. He told me that either he or I would have to go. I responded that he was the dean, so I guessed I would be the one to go. He said he would get back to me.

The next day, Dr. Kone laughed it all off. I had called his

bluff, and he blinked. But Bob had to leave. He went to Florida State, where he was the senior executive dean for many years. Months later, Dr. Kone was fired by UF for multiple issues, where he displayed a similar lack of judgment and restraint. Bob and I remain the best of friends.

GUNSHOT WOUND TO THE HEAD—TWO CASES | 22

A.K. was a distinguished professor of pathology at the University of Florida. One Wednesday afternoon, I sat and chatted with him over lunch in the faculty dining room. We talked of the usual things—the weather, medical center politics, a planned vacation. The next morning, I was summoned to the emergency room. A deranged graduate student, distraught over his failure to pass his written qualifying exams, had appeared at the professor's door early that morning. The professor's wife answered, and the student asked for the professor. When the professor appeared at the door, the student shot him in the head. The student then sat down and waited for the police and ambulance to arrive.

When I examined the professor, he was brain dead. There was nothing that I or anyone else could do, except to try to comfort the family. I paraphrase R. Selzer:

I wiped a piece of brain from the professor's shoulder, to make his smashed body more presentable to his son. Then I stood with his son by the stretcher. We were arm in arm, like brothers. All at once, there was that terrible silence of discovery. I glanced at the son, followed his gaze, and saw that there was more brain on his father's shoulder, newly slipped from the cracked skull. He bent forward a bit. He had to make certain. It was his father's brain! I watched the knowledge expand on his face, so like his father's. I, too, stared at the fragment flung wetly, now drying beneath the bright lights of the emergency room, its cargo of thoughts evaporating from it, mingling for this little time with his, with mine, before dispersing in the air (Selzer, 1976).

Here's another case—much more famous, although the details may be new to many readers. So famous, yes, but the reaction of Lincoln's doctors reads a lot like my own:

April 14, 1865, was the fourth anniversary of the surrender of Fort Sumter, in Charleston Harbor. The former fort commander, Major Robert Anderson, had been sent by President Lincoln to raise the Union flag over the ruined fort, and to preside over a general victory celebration. April 14 was also Good Friday. Abraham Lincoln, having just guided the United States through what would remain the bloodiest conflict in its entire history, did not know that this would be the last day of his life. Or did he?

Three days before his assassination, Abraham Lincoln related a dream he had to his wife and a few friends. According to Ward Hill Lamon, one of the friends who was present for the conversation, the president said:

About ten days ago, I retired very late. I had been up waiting for important dispatches from the front. I could not have been long in bed when I fell into a slumber, for I was weary. I soon began to dream. There seemed to be a death-like stillness about me. Then I heard subdued sobs, as if a number of people were weeping. I thought I left my bed and wandered downstairs. There the silence was broken by the same pitiful sobbing. No living person was in sight, but the same mournful sounds of distress met me as I passed along. I saw light in all the rooms; every object was familiar to me; but where were all the people who were grieving as if their hearts would break? I was puzzled and alarmed. What could be the meaning of all this?

Determined to find the cause of a state of things so mysterious and so shocking, I kept on until I arrived at the East Room, which I entered. There I met with a sickening surprise. Before me was a catafalque, on which rested a corpse wrapped in funeral vestments. Around it were stationed soldiers who were acting as guards; and there was a throng of people, gazing mournfully upon the corpse, whose face was covered, others weeping pitifully. 'Who is dead in the White House?' I demanded of one of the soldiers. 'The president,' was his answer; 'he was killed by an assassin.'

Then came a loud burst of grief from the crowd, which woke me from my dream. I slept no more that night; and although it was only a dream, I have been strangely annoyed by it ever since (Friedman and Peace, 2000).

Unbeknownst to the victorious Union, John Wilkes Booth, a twenty-five-year-old actor, and a band of conspirators had planned for some time to kidnap Lincoln from Ford's Theatre and take him to Virginia to force a prisoner exchange. The group's first effort failed on January 18, when Lincoln failed to show at the theater. The band, particularly John Arnold, refused to participate in a second attempt at Ford's Theatre. On March 20, they planned to kidnap Lincoln as he rode in his carriage to attend a performance of *Still Waters Run Deep* at the soldiers' home. Once again, the plot was thwarted when the president did not show.

Three of the conspirators—Arnold, Michael O'Loughlin, and John Surratt—quit in frustration and disgust at that point. However, Booth would never quit. He learned that the president and General Grant were scheduled to attend Ford's Theatre on April 14 to see the British comedy, *Our American Cousin.* He determined to assassinate the president himself that evening. He assigned Lewis Powell, a confederate veteran of many battles, to kill the secretary of state, William Seward.

Shortly after 10:00 p.m., Powell and David Herold arrived at the Seward home, the "Old Clubhouse" in Lafayette Park across from the White House. Powell gained entrance to the secretary's residence by telling the butler, William H. Bell, that he had medicine for Seward from Dr. Tullio Suzzara Verdi. (Seward, sixty-three, was quite ill due to a carriage accident and was confined to his bed in his third-floor bedroom.) Powell was well-armed. He carried an 1858 Whitney revolver, which was a large, heavy, and popular gun during the Civil War. Additionally, he carried a huge silver-mounted Bowie knife with an alligator motif and the engraving "The Hunter's Companion—Real Life Defender."

After pistol-whipping Seward's son, Frederick, Powell attacked the secretary of state with his knife. He placed his left hand on Seward's chest and then struck down with his knife several times. One stab wound went entirely through the secretary's right cheek. Although Seward was seriously injured in the attack, the leather-covered iron brace around his neck and jaw may have saved his life. In all, Powell injured five people during his wild rampage in the Seward home.

Booth instructed George Atzerodt, a carriage maker, to shoot the vice president, Andrew Johnson. Whether Atzerodt ever really agreed to do this is unproven. Whatever the case, before 8:00 a.m. on April 14, 1865, Atzerodt rented room 126 at the Kirkwood House, directly above where Johnson was staying. (The Kirkwood House was torn down after the Civil War; an office building now stands at the site on the northeast corner of 12th Street and Pennsylvania Avenue.) Atzerodt quizzed the Kirkwood House's bartender, Michael Henry, about the vice president's character and habits. However, he made no attempt on the life of Andrew Johnson. (At his trial, Atzerodt's lawyer said, "Atzerodt was guzzling like a Falstaff at 10:15 p.m.") After Lincoln's assassination, Detective John Lee found a series of incriminating items in Atzerodt's rented room (maybe planted there by Booth or David Herold).

Lincoln held a cabinet meeting that afternoon, during which he indicated his strong desire to pursue a lenient reconstruction course with the defeated Confederacy. After the meeting, General Grant told the president that he and Mrs. Grant had decided to travel on to Burlington, New Jersey, to see their children. It is possible that Mrs. Grant was trying to avoid another encounter with Mary Todd Lincoln, who had severely embarrassed her during a recent visit to the Richmond area. The Lincolns invited Major Henry Rathbone and his fiancée, Clara Harris, daughter of a senator.

After arriving at the presidential box, the president's bodyguard for the evening, John Parker, immediately deserted his post outside the box for a beer. The president's friend and longtime personal bodyguard, Ward Lamon, had reluctantly departed to Richmond as a presidential envoy. Lamon, for several years, had been nearly consumed by his fear of an assassination attempt and had frequently slept in the hallway outside the president's room at the White House.

Booth timed his entry to the presidential box to coincide with a moment of loud laughter in the play when Asa Trenchard says, "Well, I guess I know enough to turn you inside out, you sockdoligizing old man-trap." At 10:15 p.m., Booth fired his .44 derringer at Lincoln's head, slashed Rathbone with his knife, and leaped onto the stage. He caught his spur on the flag bunting and landed poorly, breaking his left leg. He shouted, "Sic semper tyrannis (thus always to tyrants)," the Virginia state motto.

Booth made his way out of the theater and escaped on horseback, later meeting up with David Herold. He was forced to alter his escape plans because of increasing pain from his broken leg. He traveled to the farm of Dr. Samuel Mudd, who cut off Booth's boot, splinted his leg, and sheltered him for half a day.

The audience at Ford's Theatre heard Mrs. Lincoln scream and saw a cloud of blue smoke emanate from the presidential box. Charles A. Leale, a twenty-three-year-old surgeon, was the first physician to reach the president. He thought he had been stabbed like Rathbone, but eventually located the gunshot entry wound. "His wound is mortal. It is impossible for him to recover." He felt the president would not survive the six-block trip to the White House. Accordingly, the unconscious president was borne from the theater across the street to the Peterson boarding house, where he was laid diagonally on a bed that was too small for him. An eight-hour deathwatch commenced.

Medical observers noted stertorous breathing, a pulse of forty-four, a dilated right pupil, left facial twitching, right facial bruising, and bulging of the right eye. Later, Lincoln had increasingly loud breathing, interrupted by complete pauses in breathing. These signs are all now known to correlate with increased intracranial pressure and brain herniation. Abraham Lincoln died at 7:22 a.m. Surgeon General Barnes placed two silver half-dollars on the president's eyes. Edwin Stanton, secretary of war, said, "Now he belongs to the ages."

After President Abraham Lincoln passed away on the morning of April 15, 1865, his body was returned by hearse to the White House. Accompanied by an escort of cavalry, the solemn procession slowly moved up 10th Street to G Street and thence to the White House. Mr. Lincoln's temporary coffin was wrapped in an American flag. His remains were transported to the guest room that was on the second floor at the front right-hand corner of the building (northwest corner). Nine men were present for the autopsy. These included Surgeon General Dr. Joseph K. Barnes; Lincoln family physician Dr. Robert King Stone; Dr. Charles Sabin Taft; Assistant Surgeon General Dr. Charles H. Crane; Army Assistant Surgeon William Morrow Notson; General Rucker of the army's Quartermaster Department (whose men had escorted the hearse back to the White House); Lincoln's friend, Orville H. Browning; Army Assistant Surgeon (pathologist) J. Janvier Woodward; and Army Assistant Surgeon (pathologist) Edward Curtis. During the necropsy, Mary Todd Lincoln sent a messenger to request a lock of hair, and a tuft was clipped from the head for her.

The actual work of the autopsy was done by Dr. Curtis and Dr. Woodward. Dr. Curtis' informal description of the autopsy (in a letter to his mother) is as follows:

The room ... contained but little furniture: a large, heavily curtained bed, a sofa or two, bureau, wardrobe, and chairs comprised all there was. Seated around the room were several general officers and some civilians, silent or conversing in whispers, and to one side, stretched upon a rough framework of boards and covered only with sheets and towels, lay—cold and immovable—what but a few hours before was the soul of a great nation. The Surgeon General was walking up and down the room when I arrived and detailed me the history of the case. He said that the President showed most wonderful tenacity of life, and, had not his wound been necessarily mortal, might have survived an injury to which most men would succumb ...

Dr. Woodward and I proceeded to open the head and remove the brain down to the track of the ball. The latter had entered a little to the left of the median line at the back of the head, had passed almost directly forwards through the center of the brain and lodged. Not finding it readily, we proceeded to remove the entire brain, when, as I was lifting the latter from the cavity of the skull, suddenly the bullet dropped out through my fingers and fell, breaking the solemn silence of the room with its clatter, into an empty basin that was standing beneath. There it lay upon the white china, a little black mass no bigger than the end of my finger—dull, motionless and harmless, yet the cause of such mighty changes in the world's history as we may perhaps never realize.

Silently, in one corner of the room, I prepared the brain for weighing. As I looked at the mass of soft gray and white substance that I was carefully washing, it was impossible to realize that it was that mere clay upon whose workings, but the day before, rested the hopes of the nation. I felt more profoundly impressed than ever with the mystery of that unknown something which may be named 'vital spark' as well as anything else, whose absence or presence makes all the immeasurable difference between an inert mass of matter owning obedience to no laws but those covering the physical and chemical forces of the universe, and on the other hand, a living brain by whose silent, subtle machinery a world may be ruled.

The weighing of the brain ... gave approximate results only, since there had been some loss of brain substance, in consequence of the wound, during the hours of life after the shooting. But the figures, as they were, seemed to show that the brain weight was not above the ordinary for a man of Lincoln's size.

Dr. Woodward's formal report of the autopsy, written to the surgeon general, is as follows:

I have the honor to report that in obedience to your orders and aided by Assistant Surgeon E. Curtis, U.S.A., I made in your presence at 12 o'clock this morning an autopsy on the body of President Abraham Lincoln, with the following results: The eyelids and surrounding parts of the face were greatly ecchymosed and the eyes somewhat protuberant from effusion of blood into the orbits. There was a gunshot wound of the head around which the scalp was greatly thickened by hemorrhage into its tissue. The ball entered through the occipital bone about one inch to the left of the median line and just above the left lateral sinus, which it opened. It then penetrated the dura matter, passed through the left posterior lobe of the cerebrum, entered the left lateral ventricle and lodged in the white matter of the cerebrum just above the anterior portion of the left corpus striatum, where it was found. The wound in the occipital bone was quite smooth, circular in shape, with beveled edges. The opening through the internal table being larger than that through the external table. The track of the ball was full of clotted blood and contained several little fragments of bone with small pieces of the ball near its external orifice. The brain around the track was pultaceous and livid from capillary hemorrhage into its substance. The ventricles of the brain were full of clotted blood. A thick clot beneath the dura matter coated the right cerebral lobe. There was a smaller clot under the dura matter of the left side. But little blood was found at the base of the brain. Both the orbital plates of the frontal bone were fractured and the fragments pushed upwards toward the brain. The dura matter over these fractures was uninjured. The orbits were gorged with blood.

Lincoln's casket lay in state in the East Room, just as he had dreamed. Then, after a brief stay in the Capitol Rotunda, his coffin and that of his son, Willie (who had died at age eleven from typhoid fever), were placed on a special funeral train for the trip to Springfield, Illinois. The train took fourteen days. The nation poured out its grief at the many stops.

On April 26, Union cavalry trapped Booth and Herold in a Virginia tobacco barn. Herold surrendered. The troops had orders to take Booth alive. Secretary Stanton suspected a widespread Confederate conspiracy. They set the barn on fire to drive him out. Despite orders, Sergeant Boston Corbett shot Booth in the back of the neck, rendering him quadriplegic. "Tell my mother I died for my country," Booth said. Looking at his hands, he said, "Useless ... useless." Then he died.

Eight conspirators were eventually tried and convicted by a special military tribunal. Edman Spangler, the stagehand who held Booth's horse, was sentenced to eight years in prison. Michael O'Loughlin, Samuel Mudd, and Samuel Arnold were sentenced to life in prison and sent to Fort Jefferson in the Dry Tortugas. O'Loughlin died there from yellow fever. Spangler, Mudd, and Arnold were pardoned in 1869 by Andrew Johnson. Although the popular view is that Mudd was innocent, the majority of historians believe that he was guilty and that his name "is still Mudd."

John Surratt escaped to Canada and Europe. He was eventually returned, was tried in a civil court, and was found innocent. Lewis Powell, George A. Atzerodt, David E. Herold, and Mary Surratt were sentenced to be hanged. On July 7, they were executed. Powell cried out that Mary Surratt was innocent and didn't deserve to die. Atzerodt said, "Goodbye, gentlemen. May we all meet in the other world."

Of course, we all know of the Lincoln Memorial, but perhaps you may not remember the words inscribed above his great statue: "In this temple, as in the hearts of his countrymen, for whom he saved the Union, the memory of Abraham Lincoln is enshrined forever."

BUMPS IN THE ROAD | 23

You've got to suffer if you want to sing the blues.
—David Bromberg

Assault by Tuna Fish

Thursday is my main day to see outpatients. Typically, I will see about twenty new patients and fifteen returns. As neurosurgery clinics go, it's a busy day. So, I got into the habit of buying lunch for everyone—the secretaries, the nurses, the residents, etc. One otherwise unremarkable Thursday, we ordered sandwiches from Jimmy John's. I specifically asked L, who was calling in the order, to make sure the med student who was working with me that day got a sandwich. About ninety minutes later, the sandwiches showed up, missing one for the med student. I should have shrugged it off, but instead, I tossed my sandwich, underhanded, to L, told her I didn't want it, said a few unkind words, and went back to my work.

A week later I was called into the senior associate dean's office. L had gone to Shands' Human Resources (HR) and complained about my behavior. She claimed I had hurled the sandwich at her. HR was going to interview all concerned. I admitted that I should have ignored the whole thing, and I apologized to L and to the other members of the clinic staff. Problem solved? No.

Several weeks later I was approached in my office by a University of Florida policewoman. She asked me to close the door. She read me the following statement, "You have the right to remain silent. Anything you say can and will be used against you in a court of law. You have the right to have an attorney. If you cannot afford one, one will be appointed to you by the court. With these rights in mind, are you still willing to talk with me about the charges against you?"

I had been Mirandized! Well, I guess there's a first time for everything. L had gone to the police and accused me of "assault." I was now being investigated.

Needless to say, I was shocked. I went to see the dean, and he suggested that we sit down with the College of Medicine attorney. She advised me to retain a personal attorney. So, I called an old friend, Judge Larry Turner. I described the entire incident to him and his assistant. He assured me that my actions could in no way be construed as assault. He encouraged me to go ahead with my scheduled trip as a visiting professor at the Dartmouth Department of Neurosurgery. I did.

When I got back, Larry called me. The UF policewoman had pursued her own investigation. That included finding the Jimmy John's delivery boy who, unbeknownst to me, had witnessed the whole thing. He confirmed my story that I had gently tossed the sandwich to L. UF police dropped the charges and the investigation.

Now back to the UF/Shands process. The associate

dean set up a meeting with me, L, and her husband. L came into the room wailing, shrieking, and otherwise incommunicative. It was quite a show, I guess intended to demonstrate that she was suffering from extreme posttraumatic stress syndrome. Her husband was indignant. Although totally nonplussed by her semi-psychotic behavior, I again apologized.

Several weeks later, I received a letter of reprimand from the dean. Basically, he said that although my version of the story had been corroborated by the investigation, if "I ever did it again" there could be severe consequences. If I ever did what again? Tossed a tuna-fish sandwich? No, he probably meant do anything remotely unkind to UF Health employees. I get it, and I buy it. At this point in my career, I am a total devotee of the team concept. It's impossible to achieve the best in medicine without creating a team. I have worked hard to mold our one hundred and seventy neurosurgery employees into something resembling a loving family. But even loving families have an occasional spat, right? What about proportionality? Shouldn't the punishment be proportional to the severity of the offense? Well, not according to most current university HR systems.

Let me tell you a couple of other stories to illustrate this point:

The X affair

About five years into my chairmanship, the dean approached me. Orthopedic surgery was trying to get rid of its adult spine surgeon, X. The dean thought he would do fine in another department and asked me, as a favor, to consider taking him. My own complex spine expert, Pat Jacob, liked X and encouraged the transfer. So I did it. After some months, several things became clear. X was smart. But it turned out that X didn't really like doing surgery. In fact, he canceled surgery on several patients at the VA Hospital whom I had already examined and scheduled for treatment. X's profit/loss statement (something I gave to every surgeon monthly) was bright red. In other words, his surgical practice wasn't coming close to covering his salary and expenses. This was very unusual for the other surgeons in the department.

Now here's where it gets tricky. While X was in the department, I made the decision to try to save the hospital money by cutting down on the number of spinal instrumentation vendors. By going with one or two vendors, it would be possible to save hundreds of thousands of dollars a year, because that sole-source vendor would give us a deep discount. The overwhelming majority of the surgeons were using one company. So, I encouraged the hospital to negotiate a contract with them. I emailed the faculty with this news and told them that they were still free to use other instrumentation if indicated for a given patient but that they would have to clear it with me.

The next morning, X, who had a long-term relationship with another vendor, called to complain. Unbeknownst to me, he went to the dean's office and accused me of taking a kickback from the selected company. Of course, this was total nonsense. Neither I nor my department got anything out of this deal. One wonders what X was getting from his vendor buddies.

Months later, at my annual evaluation, the dean asked me how X was doing. I said not well and described the issue. He suggested that I should not renew him. This is a process by which nontenured faculty can be given one year's notice, without cause. I later decided to do this. I made a big mistake by failing to get the dean's signature on the letter. A week later, he called me and told me that X had accused me of "retaliating against a whistleblower." I had absolutely no idea what he was talking about because I had no idea that he had accused me of taking a kickback, therefore, apparently, qualifying him as a whistleblower.

The dean demanded that I rescind the letter of nonrenewal. He was quite angry, which, again, I didn't understand because he himself had suggested that I issue the letter. And he, not I, had known, or should have known that X was a whistleblower! In addition, human resources and the COM attorney suggested the appointment of a committee to investigate this whole thing.

So, a committee of two people was appointed. One was a urologist who happened to be X's best friend in Gainesville! The other was a senior radiologist who knew nothing regarding the way surgeons are paid, or surgical departments are run. Instead of restricting their investigation to this specific incident, they invited anyone who had a complaint about me to come forward. They interviewed me. They specifically questioned my financial rationale for the nonrenewal. Neither one seemed to understand that the chair was responsible to the dean for the department's successful financial performance and that performance was dependent on individual surgeons doing their job well. Of course, neither was a chair. Both of their departments were propped up by injections of money taken from the profitable departments in the form of "taxes" (but that is another, very long story).

I was expecting the dean to sit down with me and X to work something out. Instead, I was totally sandbagged. Without the slightest warning, I found myself in the dean's office with the senior associate dean for clinical affairs (who didn't like me—the feeling was mutual), and the new hospital CEO. The dean told me I was suspended as chair without pay for two months and that I could return or not afterwards. He said he didn't care which. I attempted to review the entire mess but found myself about as upset as I have ever been in my life. I later received a formal certified letter from UF confirming the punishment. The dean later told me that HR had wanted to fire me, but that he wouldn't allow it considering my superb performance as chair to date.

My old mentor, Al Rhoton, was appointed acting chair in my absence. My administrator, Margaret Dermott, was shocked, and later wrote me this note:

Dr. Friedman,

I would have preferred to say this to you personally, but I was so shocked yesterday over Dean Tisher's decision that I could not pull my thoughts together. I just want you to know how much I admire all you are doing for the Department of

Neurosurgery and how incredibly effective your leadership has been. With only one obvious exception the full faculty was horrified of the outcome and the Dean's decision. There should be no doubt in your mind the entire Neurosurgery Faculty is 100% with you (again, minus that one piece of shit). Let me know if there is anything we can do. On a personal level, you make my job as administrator easy and enjoyable and I appreciate all the support you give me ... now it's my turn.

The next day, the dean met with the entire neurosurgery faculty, who unanimously supported me. Here is a description of that meeting, by my friend and colleague, Frank Bova: "I just wanted to touch base. The entire faculty found this morning's meeting very distressful. None of us can imagine the gut hit you must have taken yesterday afternoon."

To be totally honest, I was about as angry as I have ever been in my life. I consulted with several attorneys, including my childhood friend, Chuck Davidow. They all pretty much said the same thing: The university had grossly violated my rights by not following any kind of due process. They had appointed a personal friend of X to head the committee. They had not allowed me the right to view or rebut any specific allegations or to confront my accusers. And, of course, I was totally innocent of retaliating against a whistleblower. I was simply trying to do the right thing for the hospital. If we went to court, the action would be reversed. But, my attorneys said, if we did that, the university would simply wait for any excuse to come after me again. And this time, it might get the due process thing right. So, I made the best of my two-month "vacation." Then I went back to work. I'm very glad I did, for the best part of my career was yet to come. But it was very difficult.

X left, on his own accord, several months later, for another university.

John Regenfuss

Nine years ago, my wonderful departmental administrator, Margaret Dermott, decided to retire. We did a national search and found John Regenfuss to replace her. John had run many academic medical departments and had moved to Austin, TX, to assist the dean in opening a new medical school. Unfortunately, a hurricane nearly wiped out the existing medical school in San Antonio, so funds for the new school were diverted. And John came to UF.

John became my right-hand man during a period of dramatic growth in UF Health Neurosurgery. We increased our clinical faculty to sixteen. We founded a world-class brain tumor research team, led by Duane Mitchell, from Duke, and brought them to UF. Eventually that research team grew to one hundred full-time scientists and staff. We opened a UF Health Neurosurgery service at ORMC, one hundred miles away, and successfully managed it over five years. The first year, I rented a condo in Orlando and spent a minimum of three days a week there. The last four years, John and I drove down every Monday for administrative meetings, as well as patient care (me). We successfully persuaded the Shands Hospital Board of Directors to build a new neuromedicine hospital and participated in every phase of its design. We tremendously grew our patient quality improvement program and hired a full-time quality director. Etc.

I found John to be incredibly hardworking. He was always in the office before I arrived at six and was almost always the last to leave. As an MBA, he was especially valuable in the management of an increasingly complex departmental budget as it grew to a $25 million/year business. I thought he was a skilled manager of people. I received no complaints about him, ever.

So, I was shocked when the new chair (I stepped down on July 1, 2018), Brian Hoh, told me that John had been accused of sexual harassment by two female employees under his supervision. Initially, HR agreed to complete the investigation within two weeks and to allow John to continue working from home. So, he continued to drive with me every Monday to our newest practice location, Halifax Hospital in Daytona Beach (Brian asked me to help with administration there for a year). Two weeks came and went. HR then demanded that John not be allowed to work from home, but simply wait, with pay, while the investigation continued.

Months later, I was allowed to read the hundred-page report. All parties who read it—Brian, I, the dean, the university attorney, John, and his attorney—thought it was a travesty. They only interviewed witnesses supplied by the accusers. They refused to interview a list of witnesses for the defense, myself included. They injected comments like "this witness was very believable" and "the defendant was evasive." They went so far as to interview one of the accusers' mothers!

Here's what it boiled down to: John was a demanding boss. He had told the accusers, with whom he was generally friendly, that their performance was lacking. Over a year's period of time, they kept written records of anything they thought they could use against him: the time he put his hand on a shoulder, the time he gave one of them a hug, the time he made a comment about an X-rated store they passed on the highway, the time he walked through the office with a ruler in hand (he was measuring, they thought he was threatening), etc. In other words, total bullshit.

HR recommended John be nonrenewed (three months' notice at this level of employment). The dean told our chair that the choice was his. I felt strongly that John's offenses were quite minor and that he did not, in any way, deserve to be nonrenewed—especially in view of his almost nine years of superb service to the department with great annual letters of evaluation. I recommended that he be reinstated, required to take some sort of personnel management course, and be put under quarterly evaluations for a year. Brian decided to go ahead with nonrenewal. Needless to say, John's absence from our department for five months, while this miscarriage of justice was being negotiated, was very harmful.

All UF Health employees deserve respect, support, and a pleasant working environment. I strive hard to remind them, as often as possible, that every one of them is a vital member of a team which comes to work every day to do something really important: take care of our patients, educate a new generation of neurosurgeons, and, through research, find new cures for neurosurgical disease.

All UF Health employees should and do have the right to protest against any behavior which they find offensive, including any kind of harassment. The best initial way to handle harassment is to simply tell someone, "Stop. You're making me uncomfortable." If that doesn't work, go to your boss and report it. If that doesn't work, go to HR. Unfortunately, a lot of folks pull the "I was afraid of retaliation card" to work their own agenda. And the HR system is hopelessly biased against the accused. You are basically guilty until proven innocent, and the HR procedures frequently don't provide the due process by which innocence could possibly be proved. Yes, the accusers have rights. But what about the rights of the accused?

IMPROVING THE QUALITY OF MEDICAL CARE | 24

In 2012, a twenty-eight-week premature male baby was born at UF Health. Like many preemies, he had some hemorrhage into the fluid cavities of the brain and developed hydrocephalus. He underwent a simple neurosurgical procedure called a ventriculoperitoneal shunt. This is a thirty-minute operation where a plastic catheter is placed in the ventricle, through a small hole in the skin, and then tunneled under the skin to an abdominal incision. The fluid that was blocked up in the brain can then travel through the tube and be reabsorbed in the abdominal cavity.

The boy did well until age two when he presented to our emergency room with episodic vomiting and lethargy. He was admitted for observation, improved, and was discharged with instructions to return to the pediatric neurosurgery clinic. Months later, he finally made it to the clinic, and a shunt malfunction was diagnosed based on a scan that showed increased ventricular size. He was scheduled for surgery the next day. That night, at home, he became suddenly comatose and was transported to the hospital where he had emergency surgery. Unfortunately, while comatose, he had herniated, which means that the brain pushed downward against the arteries that supplied his occipital cortex. As a result, he had bilateral occipital lobe strokes, which left him blind. What a disaster!

How could this happen? As after all major complications, a committee was rapidly convened to perform what we call a root-cause analysis. The root causes in this case included failure to recognize a shunt malfunction on the initial ER visit, the fact that the patient's symptoms were intermittent, the fact that the patient's mother was a nurse who thought he was fine, and the fact that the family ignored instructions to come to the ER until it was too late. In other words, as with most major medical complications, there were multiple errors. James Reason, a scholar of error mitigation, calls this "lining up the holes in the Swiss cheese." There were multiple opportunities to prevent a catastrophe, and all of them had to be missed for it to occur.

Quality improvement in medicine is a relatively recent development in medicine spurred on by the Institute of Medicine's 2000 publication, *To Err Is Human* (Institute of Medicine, 2000). In that report, they estimated that medical errors resulted in upwards of ninety-eight thousand deaths per year in the United States. They found that more people died in a given year as a result of medical errors than from motor vehicle accidents, breast cancer, or AIDS. A second publication, in 2001, *Crossing the Quality Chasm: A New Health System for the 21st Century*, provided a strategy for substantial improvement.

Although this focus is relatively new in medicine, it has been central to the commercial aviation industry for over fifty years. In the late 1930s, new military aircraft became so complex that even the best pilots were crashing them with regularity. The airline response was the development of checklists for every phase of aviation. For example, in my Cirrus SR22, there is a detailed checklist for preflight inspection; engine start, climb, cruise, descent, and landing. In addition, there is a checklist for every emergency you can think of. The airline industry has also emphasized the concept of "crew resource management," wherein the entire crew is actively encouraged to communicate any and all of their concerns immediately to the captain.

Here's an example of a rare but massive failure to use these methods properly in the aviation industry: On March 27, 1977, jets arriving in Tenerife were diverted, because of fog, to the smaller Los Rodeos Airport. KLM 4805 and Pan Am 1735 both had to taxi down the only runway and turn around for takeoff. Because of dense fog, the planes couldn't see each other, and the controllers couldn't see either plane. KLM, under the control of the chief pilot, attempted a takeoff, without clearance (!!) while Pan Am was still back-taxiing on the runway. The planes, both with full fuel, collided and burst into a fireball. All 248 people on KLM were killed, and 335 out of 396 on Pan Am were killed. It remains the worst disaster in aviation history. And it was clearly due to failure to communicate per standard procedure and, in the case of KLM, the failure of the captain to listen to his subordinates.

Here's an example of everything going right, avoiding

disaster: On January 1, 2009, Airbus A329 departed LaGuardia for Charlotte. The pilot in command was Chesley Sullenberger. His co-pilot was Jeffrey Skiles. They also had three very experienced flight attendants. Immediately after takeoff, they encountered a flock of Canadian geese that were sucked into the engines. They lost power in both engines. The captain took the controls while the copilot worked the emergency checklists of engine restart, then forced landing. After rejecting options to return to LaGuardia (later shown to fail in simulations), they ditched in the Hudson. The attendants conducted a perfect evacuation, and no lives were lost. The NTSB attributed this superb result to checklist use and excellent crew resource management.

So, can checklists work in medicine? In his book, *The Checklist Manifesto*, Harvard surgeon Atul Gawande says unequivocally, yes (Gawande, 2010). The four killers in surgery are infection, bleeding, anesthesia, and the unexpected. All are amenable to aviation-style checklist. All are amenable to improved communication, just like aviation. The most commonly employed surgical checklist today is the World Health Organization's Surgical Safety Checklist. Before the induction of anesthesia, the attending surgeon, the attending anesthesiologist, and the patient verify the patient's identity, the site and side of surgery, the precise procedure, and the signed consent. Questions about allergies, blood availability, positioning, needed equipment, and post-op plans are quickly reviewed and verified. Immediately before incision, a time-out is called for repeat verification. All personnel in the OR are introduced if they haven't worked together before. At the end of the case, a quick debriefing covers calling the family, equipment issues encountered, and disposition of surgical specimens. This checklist has been tested in hundreds of hospitals in dozens of countries and found to consistently improve surgical outcomes. Its use is now required in all US hospitals.

Modern error management recognizes that people will never stop making mistakes. Improving quality, therefore, usually involves improving systems to make it easy to do the right thing and hard to do the wrong thing. In the modern "just culture" model of patient safety there are four categories of error. The very rare "malicious error," like the nursing home attendant who dispatches his patients, requires legal action. Errors that involve an impaired practitioner, say due to alcohol, drugs, or illness, require intervention and may need restriction of practice. But the overwhelming majority of errors are "inadvertent." They require fixing the system and educating those involved in the error.

I became very interested in neurosurgical quality improvement about ten years ago. I attended the Executive Leadership course sponsored by the Institute for Healthcare Improvement in Boston and came back with a new outlook and a new set of tools. We initially focused on a high infection rate for a procedure called a ventriculostomy. A ventriculostomy is a small plastic tube usually inserted under local anesthesia at the patient's bedside. A small hole is drilled in the skull, and the tube is directed into the ventricle so that blocked-up fluid can drain into an external bag. It's like a temporary shunt.

Infected ventriculostomies lead to meningitis, which

can lead to very serious, sometimes permanent neurological issues. At a minimum, they require prolonging hospitalization for antibiotic treatment. In order to tackle the problem, we assembled a multidisciplinary team, including me, a senior resident, a nurse, an infectious disease specialist, and a quality improvement facilitator. We identified many potential root causes, including too many locations for the procedure, lack of meticulous gowning and draping, poor lighting, poor bed condition, lack of prophylactic antibiotics, and nonuse of an antibiotic-impregnated ventriculostomy catheter. We developed a checklist that we printed and laminated for all of our doctors. We enlisted the nurses in the units to monitor the use of the checklist on every ventriculostomy. Bottom line—for the past five years, after hundreds of procedures, we haven't had a single infection!

The quality improvement paradigm described above has been used on dozens of subsequent quality improvement projects in our department. Neurology and Neurosurgery have since hired a PhD-quality improvement director who oversees dozens of quality improvement projects. We have two morning conferences per month, focusing on quality improvement, reviewing every case where there is any type of complication. Equally importantly, we are preparing our faculty and residents to deal with this reality: our patients expect very high-quality care and are increasingly able to evaluate us based on publicly reported quality measures like mortality, length of stay, and infection rate by individual surgeons.

As information systems and government mandates

make our outcomes more and more transparent to the public, I believe our health-care system as a whole can become much better. Providers and institutions will not be rewarded with more money for doing more procedures; they will be rewarded with more patients by doing fewer procedures on the right patients, with better outcomes!

HOW DOCTORS THINK (OR DON'T) | 25

An expert is someone who learns more and more about less and less until he knows everything about nothing.
—Nicholas Butler

spent the first two weeks of March 2020 visiting my friend and colleague, Doug Kondziolka, at New York University. Doug is a world-renowned expert in radio-surgery, using a device called the gamma knife. Although I specialized in radiosurgery using a different device, the linear accelerator (see chapter 15), I had never actually seen the gamma knife in use. Over the course of the visit, I learned a lot from Doug, and he learned a bit, I think, from me as well. And, of course, I had a great time in the Big Apple, enjoying restaurants, plays, and opera.

About a week after I returned to Gainesville, I felt chilled and achy. I had a low-grade fever. I also had right-sided chest pain, made worse by breathing (that's called pleuritic chest pain). Of course, everyone, including my doctor, Heather Harrell, was focused on COVID. So, I self-quarantined and got a COVID test, which was negative. My symptoms resolved and, a week later, I was allowed to return to work.

All was well, until ten days later when the chills and

low-grade fever returned. This time the right-sided pleuritic chest pain was so bad, I couldn't believe it. I wound up going to the emergency room at 4 a.m. Although my vital signs were okay, and another COVID test was negative, they were concerned about the severe chest pain. A CT angiogram of my chest revealed a large, right-sided pulmonary embolus. Pulmonary emboli are life-threatening blood clots that form in the lungs and make it difficult to breathe. They also are well known to cause pleuritic chest pain. The treatment is blood thinners to prevent further clots, usually for months or years. I was admitted, anticoagulated, and discharged feeling much better. Again, I returned to work.

How could this happen? How could very good physicians (myself included) focus totally on COVID to the exclusion of other diagnoses and miss a potentially lethal problem? Well, it turns out that we are hardwired to make just this kind of mistake, not only in medicine but in many other walks of life. My resident colleague, Kyle Fargen, and I reviewed these built-in errors in a paper many years ago (Fargen and Friedman, 2014).

The process of analytical medical decision-making ideally involves a series of cognitive steps. These progress through outlining the goal and desired outcome; comprehending the problem at hand; evaluating available choices and developing alternatives; considering the pros and cons of each option; making the decision; taking action to implement the decision; and finally, learning from and reflecting on the decision that was generated. However, this stepwise process is used for only a fraction of the decisions that are made by physicians during any given day. Frequently, major decisions are made rapidly and subconsciously, bypassing this complex analytical series of steps.

Rapid decisions generated from nonanalytical cognition are highly influenced by previous experiences and the outcomes that were obtained in similar situations (biases), even though patients often have highly variable symptoms and signs. A number of important cognitive biases that invariably impede accurate physician decision-making have been identified. The two different decision-generation processes (analytical and nonanalytical) have recently been explained by dual-process theory (DPT).

DPT asserts that humans developed two separate and distinct processes of reasoning during evolution. System 1, or the implicit system, is the process by which automatic decisions are generated rapidly through intuition, unconscious reasoning, and previous experiences and memories. System 2, or the explicit system, is a higher-order process that allows for conscious reasoning with judgments based on critical examination. System 2 is slow and tedious, is influenced by logic and evidence, operates only with effort, and may overcome decisions generated in System 1.

It is argued that we spend approximately 95 percent of the time behaving intuitively. Many of these intuitive judgments are aided by heuristics—mental rules, shortcuts, and maxims. Although heuristics allow for rapid decision-making, they are subject to considerable biases and error. Integral to our understanding of how diagnostic errors occur is the recognition of the most common biases:

Anchoring – The tendency to weigh initial data too heavily during the diagnostic process and failure to adapt once more information is available. That's what happened to me—everyone "anchored" on COVID.

Availability bias – The tendency to judge diagnoses as more likely if they were recently seen. Ditto.

Commission bias – The tendency to promote patient beneficence through action rather than inaction.

Confirmation bias – The tendency to look for evidence to confirm that diagnosis rather than look for evidence to refute it.

Diagnosis momentum – The tendency for an initial diagnosis to gain traction.

Fundamental attribution error – The tendency to blame patients for their situation or illness.

Overconfidence bias – The tendency of individuals to believe that they are more knowledgeable than they actually are.

Search satisfying – The tendency to stop looking for other problems once one is identified.

Visceral bias – Decisions are more likely to be poor when the clinician is emotionally labile.

There are many more biases. I have seen them all and have committed them all many times.

De-biasing begins with becoming aware of our own biases. As discussed in the chapter on quality improvement, physicians are profoundly affected by complications they cause. A good quality improvement program uses this motivation to teach bias avoidance. Other useful strategies include using algorithms when possible. Controlling for overconfidence. Ruling out worst-case scenarios. Recognizing emotion and fatigue. Discussing diagnoses and treatments with colleagues. Above all, always think to yourself, "Am I making a mistake?"

I have made way too many.

WAF

REFERENCE LIST

Chalmers, David. *Explaining Consciousness: The Hard Problem*. Cambridge, MA: MIT Press, 1996.

Csikszentmihalyi, Mihaly. *Flow: The Psychology of Optimal Experience*. New York: Harper & Row, 1990.

Dreyfus, Stuart E., and Hubert L. Dreyfus. *A Five-Stage Model of the Mental Activities Involved in Directed Skill Acquisition*. Berkeley: Operations Research Center, University of California, Berkeley, 1980.

Ericsson, K. A., and W. Kintsch. "Long-Term Working Memory." *Psychological Review* 102 (1995): 211–45.

Fargen, K., and W. Friedman. "The Science of Medical Decision Making: Neurosurgery Errors and Personal Cognitive Strategies for Improving Quality of Care." *World Neurosurgery* 82 (2014): 21–29.

Frankl, Viktor. *Man's Search for Meaning: An Introduction to Logotherapy*. Boston: Beacon Press, 2006 (first edition 1959).

Friedman, W., and D. Peace. "A Gunshot Wound to the Head—the Case of Abraham Lincoln." *Surgical Neurology* 53 (2000): 511–15.

Gawande, Atul. *Checklist Manifesto: How to Get Things Right.* New York: Metropolitan Books, 2010.

Gunther, John. *Death Be Not Proud: A Memoir.* New York: Modern Library, 1953.

Institute of Medicine (US) Committee on Quality of Health Care in America, L. T. Kohn, J. M. Corrigan, M. S. Donaldson, eds. *To Err Is Human: Building a Safer Health System.* Washington, DC: National Academies Press (US), 2000.

Institute of Medicine (US) Committee on Quality of Health Care in America. *Crossing the Quality Chasm: A New Health System for the 21st Century.* Washington, DC: National Academies Press (US), 2001.

Jackson, Frank. "What Mary Didn't Know." *The Journal of Philosophy* 83, no. 5 (May 1986): 291–95.

Searle, John. "Minds, Brains, and Programs." *The Behavioral and Brain Sciences* 3 (1980): 417–24.

Selzer, Richard. *Mortal Lessons: Notes on the Art of Surgery.* New York: Simon & Schuster, 1976.

Solzhenitsyn, Aleksandr. *Cancer Ward.* New York: Dial Press, 1968.